TREASURES OF HEALTH

NUTRITION
MANUAL

TREASURES OF HEALTH

NUTRITION MANUAL

DISCOVER THE ANSWERS TO ALL YOUR HEALTH QUESTIONS

ANNETTE REEDER
AND
DR. RICHARD COUEY

designed publishing

ISBN 13: 978-0-9853969-1-6
ISBN 10: 1-4141-1725-6
Library of Congress Catalog Card Number: 2010901623

Author's Note

Health is a gift not to be taken for granted. It is affected by diet, accidents, stress, pollution and lifestyle. The information contained in this book is not designed to treat disease nor cure any illness, but rather to help you learn how disease may originate from nutritional deficiencies. As a Christian we are called to live a disciplined healthy life. When it comes to our health, following the guidelines expressed in the Bible leads to greater health but many times our shortcomings are a result of uninformed choices and lack of discipline.

To appreciate the gift given to you, learn all you can about your health and how to protect it. Always consult your physician in regards to your medical care and medications. This book does not replace the advice of your physician.

These statements have not been evaluated by the Food and Drug Administration. This information is not intended to diagnose, treat, cure or prevent any disease.

CONTENTS

CONTENTS

Our Mental Health

Our Spiritual Health

CONTENTS

Resources

MY WORD OF THANKS

My partner, co-author and content advisor: Dr. Couey has a heart for missions and missionaries. His desire to see them stay healthy and continue going forth made writing this book with his expertise a delight. It is his desire and mine to take this message forward to many missionaries and mission sending agencies around the globe.

My contributing authors: Dr. Stephen G. Chaney, Dr. Richard Brouse, Bonnie Morrell, and Martha Wilmore. Their contributions to health education and the gracious notes for this book made this more complete.

It is difficult to see only two names on the book when there have been a team of people making this happen. Without the fellowship of these friends and colleagues, this book would never be in your hands.

For You

This book was written for you, the one looking for a composite collection of nutrition answers. This nutrition manual is a must to have within reach for all your questions about health. Add this book to your collection of the *Treasures of Healthy Living* Bible study and the *Healthy Treasures* cookbook and you have a trio of applicable tools to give you guidance for years to come.

INTRODUCTION: IF ONLY I HAD KNOWN

HAVE YOU EVER heard yourself say, "If only I had known"? Do you then add: "I could have made better decisions"; "I could have made better investments"; "I could have used my time differently"; or "I could have avoided that situation"? How many times could *knowing* have helped you avoid tripping over a rock, buying the wrong garment, buying a lemon of a car, traveling down the wrong road, losing your car keys, or eating unhealthy food? If only you had known of the waterfall waiting at the end, you could have hiked a beautiful trail; or if you had known more, you could have worked a little harder to achieve the ultimate reward.

Hosea 4:6 tells us, "My people are destroyed for lack of knowledge." If the people in Hosea's time had only known or understood what the genuinely concerned prophet was trying to teach them they could have repented and experienced love, forgiveness and refreshing healing. Today we have an even greater Prophet teaching us the way to live our lives. Our prophet is Christ Himself. Colossians 2:2–3 says, "…their hearts may be encouraged, having been knit together in love, and attaining to all the wealth that comes from the full assurance of understanding, resulting in a true knowledge of God's mystery, that is Christ Himself, in whom are hidden all the treasures of wisdom and knowledge." From Christ's teachings we can reverse the phrase, "If only I had known," to "now I know." What better teacher would you prefer to have?

Now, we know that Scripture is an abundant treasure chest full of blessings to our health. This book, along with two companions, *Treasures of Healthy Living Bible Study* and *Healthy Treasures Cookbook*, will elaborate on those and direct you to the knowledge and understanding of how God designed your body, what foods are going to deliver nutrition, the value of vitamins, and the ultimate treasure of being happy and healthy.

In my family, we now say, "Now I know." We know how to dip into this treasure and work to protect against problems like cancer, pre-diabetes, high blood pressure, Osgood Slater's disease, irritable bowel syndrome, "growing pains," dental problems, allergies, being overweight, and many others issues plaguing America today. Now we know God's foods make a difference. Now we know there is a better way to live.

I must confess, this knowing and applying is a daily choice and not every day is spent in perfect harmony. There are still many times when cookies, ice cream or laziness call my name. The difference is now I know that my body is on loan to me to fulfill a purpose. I know there are better choices to make.

Many times people say, "If only I had known," and then don't make any changes. Today you can change. In this book are numerous steps to make healthy changes for yourself and your family.

Dr. Couey and I have compiled an encyclopedia of information for you to treasure for years to come and to help you achieve the highest level of health available under the Son.

Join us in changing your tune to "I am glad that *now I know*." Knowledge and application from God's Word generates years of health and a treasure full of wonderful memories as you gain vitality and fulfillment.

Now I know and you can know too as we claim this verse: "In Him you have been made complete" Colossians 2:10.

WHY SHOULD CHRISTIANS BE HEALTHY?

You created my inmost being; You knit me together in my mother's womb. I praise you because I am fearfully and wonderfully made.

Psalm 139:1 NIV

God's Greatest Creation

THE GENESIS ACCOUNT of creation reveals that God's creation of man and woman was His greatest. He created man in His image and likeness (Gen. 1:26), and He breathed in him the breath of life (Gen. 2:7). The Scriptures disclose that God was very proud of this creation: "God saw all that He had made, and behold, it was very good" (Gen. 1:31). Just as we marvel and take pride in things that we do well, so God does marvel and take pride in what He created so perfectly.

Fearfully and Wonderfully Made

As a physiologist, one who studies the functions of the human body, I am amazed at how complicated, intricate, and diversified is each part and system in the body, yet how each lives in such harmony, efficiently performing specific tasks. To me, the human body is perhaps the supreme wonder of the universe.

For example, let us look at some of the marvels of the body as God created it:

- You build a trillion cells a day by what you eat.
- There are 80–100 trillion cells in your body.
- The body will produce approximately 2–10 million red blood cells each second of your life.
- By the time you can count to ten, the blood in your veins and arteries has traveled

more than 12,000 miles.
- Every single person who is living and ever has lived has different shaped fingerprints.
- The nerve cells carry messages to and from the brain at speeds faster than a 38-calliber pistol shot.
- It takes 19 vitamins and minerals and 9 amino acids with a perfect protein to build a perfect cell—even if you only miss 1 nutrient, then you are building imperfect cells for 7 days. These defective cells will promote the development of degenerative diseases. You are the only one who can do something about it!

With proper consumption, assimilation, and elimination, our bodies have the ability to change:

- The chemistry of the blood in seven days.
- The composition of cells in seven weeks.
- Some major organs in seven months.

In addition:

- As science knows, have a completely new body in seven years.
- Physiological chemists state that there is not a blood cell more than 14 days old, and that we rebuild a new heart every 30 days.

After reading this list, is there any wonder why God called his creation "good"? To experience the good, we must examine our lifestyles, whether it is our mental, spiritual, emotional, or physical development, and analyze how they can affect the chemistry of our cells. If we neglect our development in these four areas, then our cells' chemistry will be compromised and illness can be encountered. For illness to be prevented or cured, then our cell's chemistry must be restored to God's intended design. Once our cells' chemistry is normal, then the cells can repair themselves. *Health and healing begin at the cellular level.*

God Owns Our Bodies

God made man in "His own image" (Gen. 1:27), and that man became a living person. The first man was in a state of physical perfection. Every system in this body, including every cell, was in perfect working condition. This was the ultimate in physical fitness. There was no air pollution; noise pollution; junk food; or automatic, labor-saving devices to mar this perfection. One can almost sense the awe that God felt as he viewed His wonderful creation and said that "it was *very* good" (Gen. 1:31, italics mine).

God knows every minute detail about our bodies. Under the inspiration of the Holy Spirit,

Paul wrote, "What, know ye not that your body is the temple of the Holy Spirit which is in you, which ye have of God, and ye are not your own? For ye are bought with a price: therefore glorify God in your body, and in your spirit, which are God's" (1 Cor. 6:19–20, KJV).

This scripture clearly reveals that your body does not belong to you. Examine these verses again. "Know ye not that your body is the temple of the Holy Spirit…which ye have of God, and ye are not your own? For ye are bought with a price." God created your body in His likeness. He breathed the breath of life into it. And He paid a great price in proving His love for you and redeeming you from sin. If you are a professing Christian, you have greater reason than others to take care of your body until you take your last breath. For Christians, care of the body is a matter of stewardship. A steward, as defined by Webster, refers to a supervisor who manages an estate of property for someone else. God has given us bodies, and He expects us to feed, rest, and exercise them properly, and to grow in both mind and spirit. He wants us to use our bodies to give glory to Him, because He owns them. If we do not keep our bodies in the best possible physical condition, they are incapable of honoring God as they should.

There is no set number of years at which we can say we are old. Old age is simply a degeneration of the body brought about by wrong feeding and living habits. Remember, no matter how many years you have lived, there is not a cell in the body more than seven years old.

Therefore, as professing Christians and good stewards, we have the responsibility to carefully maintain internally and externally the temples that God created. We should continually and consistently develop our bodies mentally, emotionally, spiritually, and physically for the best possible performance and production capability.

To help you achieve this performance, this nutrition manual is divided up into three parts. Part 1 will teach you about the foods gifted to us by God for our health. After reading it, you too may be called "Nuts about Nutrition." Part 2 will give you guidance on the value of vitamins, which foods contain them, and how to find healthy supplements. Part 3 will give you instructions on how to prevent and overcome health challenges using the nutrition tools as a guide. With all of these together, you now have in your hands a huge resource manual to give you guidance for years to come and to help you live a life that is glorifying to God in all areas.

A SAMPLE DAY— TREASURES OF HEALTHY LIVING

Great are the works of the Lord, they are studied by all who delight in them.

Psalm 111:2

WHAT DOES A healthy day of eating look like? Many people through the years of classes have asked this question so here is a sample schedule for you to use as a basis for your own personal plan. Obviously times and foods will vary but this is a general starting point.

Daily Schedule for Healthy Living:

6:00	Wake up and drink two cups of water with freshly squeezed organic lemons or herbal tea.
6:00–7:00	Spend time in prayer, Bible study, and worship. Some will need to limit this to get things ready for their families, but at least thirty minutes of worship time will yield the best day.
7:00	Breakfast: 50% fresh fruits, flax seed, and yogurt or a protein shake. Limit juice, unless it is made fresh. Fresh-milled bread would be a good addition.
8:00–9:00	Twenty to sixty minutes of exercise.
9:00–11:30	Sometime between two hours after breakfast and one half-hour before lunch, drink two eight-ounce glasses of water.
12:00	Lunch: 50% raw veggies, protein and fresh milled bread. Fruits allowed.
2:00–5:30	Between meals, drink two eight-ounce glasses of water.
Afternoon	Enjoy at least ten minutes, in all seasons, for a time of fresh air and sunshine. Breathe deeply while outside.

6:00	Dinner: Power 5 Salad – a salad made with at least 5 ingredients including your choice of: beans, greens, vegetables, fruit, seeds, and nuts. Add to this high quality protein.
7:30	Drink two glasses of water.
9:30	Begin winding down.
10:00	Bedtime

As you follow this example or design one for yourself, remember that it is for the health of your body that you are following this plan. Make a list of dreams God has placed on your heart that you could accomplish if health problems were not taking yours or your family's time and energy.

Behold, to obey is better than sacrifice.

1 Samuel 15:22

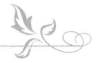

PART 1 —
NUTS ABOUT NUTRITION

When you have eaten and are satisfied, you shall bless the Lord your God for the good land which He has given you.

Deuteronomy 8:10

YOU ARE WHAT you eat. Do you believe this statement? Does that mean a health nut is someone who eats a lot of nuts? I think there is more to us than just what we eat. But nutrition plays a huge role in the energy and vitality in which we will live our lives. The study of nutrition and God's design deserves our time so that we can live productive lives until we reach heaven, not just until we retire.

Are you ready to understand the foods gifted to us by a loving God? Are you ready to see which foods will build health? Nuts about Nutrition gives the information needed to make good healthy decisions on foods to buy and foods to avoid. Since everything we consume affects our health, it's time to understand food's value. Have fun exploring new foods and finding unique favorites. Don't let past experiences detour you on this journey.

Tools for the Journey

There are 320,000 edible items for sale on a typical day in the United States. Most suburban grocery stores carry as many as 40,000 of these items. Do you have a plan for finding food that will build health? Do you have a measuring stick to use for making good choices? How do you decide between low-fat and heart-healthy foods?

Dr. Rex Russell's book, *What the Bible Says About Healthy Living* (Regal Publishing), led me to one of the best discoveries to help simplify shopping choices: The Three Principles. These principles form the foundation for making choices in regard to all areas of health:

- Principle 1: Eat only substances God created for food. Avoid what is not designed for food.
- Principle 2: As much as possible, eat foods as they were created—before they are changed or converted into something humans think might be better.
- Principle 3: Avoid food addictions. Don't let any food or drink become your god.

These three principles are taught extensively in the Treasures of Healthy Living Bible study. Memorizing these principles will assist you to make healthy choices.

FOODS IN THE BIBLE

All things bright and beautiful, All creatures great and small, All things wise and wonderful, The Lord God made them all.

Cecil Frances Alexander, 1818–1895

THE BIBLE IS like a cookbook." This statement came from one of our class participants after she began her journey through the *Treasures of Healthy Living Bible Study*. Truly, there are more scriptures regarding food than most people realize. Here is a short listing of some references to food in Scripture. It is helpful to read these individually over a course of time to get the full impact of God's design. When you finish this list there will be more verses in your daily reading that will inspire you regarding health and food. In the end, it is wise to remember *the Lord God made them all.*

God, the Provider[1]

Genesis 1:29
Genesis 27:28
Exodus 16
Deuteronomy 8:10–18
Psalm 85:11–12
Psalm 104:14, 27–28

Genesis 9:3
Exodus 12:1–11
Deuteronomy 12:20–25
1 Kings 17:16
Luke 22:7–8
Luke 24:41–43
John 6:11
John 21:5–13
Romans 14:6–8
1 Timothy 4:1–5

The Issue of Vegetarianism

Genesis 4:2–5

Vegetarian Diet

(As a personal choice)
Daniel 1:8–16
Proverbs 15:17
Romans 14:3–4
1 Corinthians 6:12

Meat

Genesis 9:3–4
Genesis 18:1–8
Leviticus 7:22–23, 26
Leviticus 7:28–36
Leviticus 11
Deuteronomy 14
Deuteronomy 32:14
1 Kings 4:22–23
Acts 15:22–29
John 6:11

Grains

Genesis 41:56–42:2
Deuteronomy 8:8
Deuteronomy 32:14
Ruth 2
Isaiah 28:23–29
Judges 7:13
1 Samuel 17:17
2 Kings 4:42

Food Lists

Genesis 43:11
Deuteronomy 8:7–9
Deuteronomy 32:13–14
1 Samuel 25:18
2 Samuel 17:28–29
Numbers 11:5

Honey

Numbers 14:7–8
Deuteronomy 32:13
Proverbs 24:13
Proverbs 25:16, 27
1 Samuel 14:24–29
Isaiah 7:14–15
Isaiah 7:22
Mark 1:6
Psalm 19:10

Salt

Job 6:6
Matthew 5:13
Colossians 4:6

Oil

Deuteronomy 8:8
Deuteronomy 32:13
1 Kings 17:7–16
Proverbs 21:17, 20

Butter, Curds, Cream, and Cheese

Genesis 18:1–8
Deuteronomy 32:14
Judges 5:25
Proverbs 30:33
Isaiah 7:14–15
Isaiah 7:21–22
Job 10:10
1 Samuel 17:18
2 Samuel 17:29

Milk

Genesis 18:1–8
Numbers 14:7–8
Deuteronomy 32:14
Judges 4:19
Proverbs 27:27
Isaiah 55:1
Ezekiel 25:4
Joel 3:18
1 Corinthians 4:7

Nuts

Genesis 43:11

Eggs

Job 6:6
Luke 11:11–12

Fruits and Vegetables

Genesis 25:34
Numbers 11:5
Numbers 13:23
Deuteronomy 23:24
Deuteronomy 28:40
2 Samuel 16:1–2
Ezekiel 4:9

HEALTHY TREASURES FRESH MARKET PYRAMID: YOUR KEY TO SUCCESS

WHAT DID JESUS eat? Would Mary, Jesus' mother, have shopped the market and gathered food for the day? Was there fresh fish brought in from the sea for her to purchase for her family? If scripture declares certain foods "good" then we know Jesus, his parents and siblings would have eaten these wholesome foods. What we need is a visual to remind us of the "good".

In our culture the most common visual is the food pyramid. Dieticians and physicians have given us several food pyramids, but the one with the most solid foundation—with extensive research going back fifty years—is the Mediterranean Pyramid. According to the Mayo Clinic, this pyramid has demonstrated the highest average life expectancy and the lowest rates of chronic diseases among adults.[2] People have taken notice of this diet's benefits, and now restaurants, cooking shows, and cookbooks have embraced this way of meal planning. You and your foodie friends can join in on the culinary delight.

The Mediterranean pyramid maximizes natural, whole foods and minimizes highly processed ones. Dr. Steve Parker summarizes the Mediterranean Diet Pyramid in his book *The Advanced Mediterranean Diet*: "Clinical studies have clearly shown that a Mediterranean style diet is associated with overall greater health and longevity, lower incidence of cancers, and lower incidence of cardiovascular disease. Furthermore, recent studies suggest that such a diet may reduce dementia of both Alzheimer's and vascular types. Expert consensus is that the health benefits are due to diet composition coupled with a physically active lifestyle."[3, 4] We have modified the Mediterranean pyramid by removing the foods and drinks that bring harm to the body and were declared unclean.

The Healthy Treasures Fresh Market accentuates the freshest ingredients to build a healthy diet. This is a reminder of the foods Jesus was served while he fellowshipped around the dinner table. For the Healthy Treasures Fresh Market Pyramid, we have updated the Mediterranean

Pyramid by eliminating unclean foods and categories such as herbs, grains, and vegetables have been made easy to recognize.

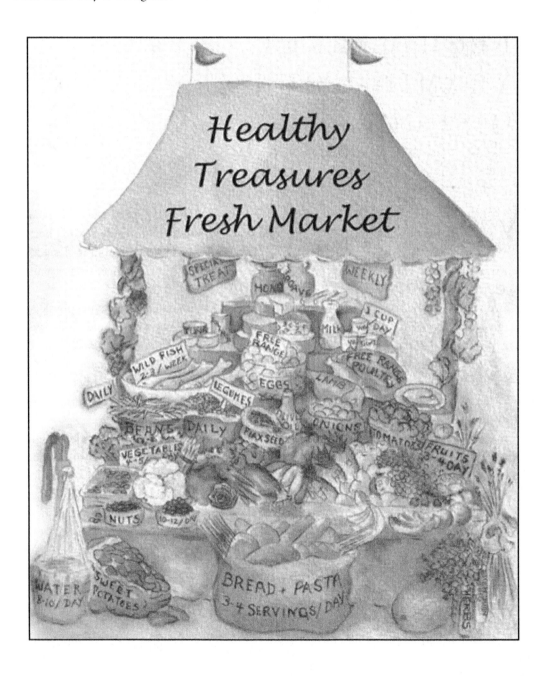

WATER AND
BEVERAGES

Everyone who drinks this water will be thirsty again, but whoever drinks the water I give him will never thirst. Indeed, the water I give him will become a spring of water welling up to eternal life.

John 4:13, 14 NIV

THE SIMPLE ELEMENTS God created continue to be our best medicines. Fresh clean air, pure water, and superior fresh foods that add fiber to the diet are the vital ingredients that help prevent many diseases. Man is still unacquainted with the numerous benefits of water. Although we love to use water for pleasure and refreshment on a hot day, if we truly understood the benefits of water, our desire for it would increase.

Consuming water can slow down the aging process. In addition, many other diseases can be prevented and/or improved by consuming quality water. Just give it a try, and you will feel the difference quickly. It is not expensive and certainly worth the effort.

For maximum benefit, you must drink one half (½) of your body weight in ounces of water daily. Here are some examples of the amounts of water people need*:

> Your weight: 150 lbs. = 75 ounce = 9 glasses of water
> 125 lbs. = 68 ounce = 8 ½ glasses of water
> 200 lbs. = 100 ounce = 12 ½ glasses of water

*Drink your water at least thirty minutes before a meal and then two hours after a meal to aid in efficient enzyme activity during digestion.

Drinking enough water has many benefits for the body. Below are listed some of the many functions of water. Water:

- Is the primary energizer of all functions in the body.
- Is the adhesive that bonds cell's membranes.
- Eliminates many bladder, bowel, and migraine problems.
- Relieves many anxiety attacks and food tolerance reactions.
- Relieves colitis pain, hot flashes, and headaches.
- Is necessary for digestion and metabolism.
- Keeps kidneys healthy.
- Helps with Chronic Fatigue Syndrome.
- Carries nutrients and oxygen to cells through the blood.
- Regulates the body temperature through perspiring.
- Helps to lubricate joints.
- Flushes out toxins.
- Enhances brain function.
- Fights obesity—helps turn the appetite switch off.
- Reduces breast cancer risk by 70%.
- Reduces colon cancer risk by 45%.
- Relieves stress.

Hydration vs. Dehydration

Hydrating drinks (in order of value)
Purified water
Tap water
Bottled water
Juice—fresh-squeezed is best
Herbal teas, non-caffeine
Milk and non-milk—soy, rice, almond
Carbonated soda w/o caffeine

Dehydrating drinks
coffee
tea—caffeinated
beer
wine
all other alcoholic drinks
carbonated soda w/ caffeine

Daily our goal should be to drink the appropriate amount of water for our bodies. When we drink eight glasses of water and then in the same day drink one caffeinated soda and two cups of caffeinated tea, we have just cancelled out three of the eight glasses of water. Every six ounces of caffeine or alcohol requires an additional ten to twelve ounces of water to rehydrate you.

The 10 Commandments of Good Hydration[5]

1. Drink 1/2 ounce daily for every pound you weigh.
2. Avoid diuretic beverages that flush water out of your body, such as caffeinated coffee, tea, soda, alcohol, and beer.
3. Drink more water and fresh juices to maintain hydration during illness and upon recovery. Illness robs your body of water.
4. Start your day with 1/2 to 1 quart of water to flush your digestive tract and rehydrate your system from the overnight fast.
5. Drink water at regular intervals throughout the day. Don't wait until you're thirsty.
6. Get in the habit of carrying a water bottle with you. Keep one in the car or on your desk. Convenience helps. Use a water purifier in your home and refill a quality bottle to go with you.
7. Make a habit of drinking water. Decide to drink before every meal—at least 30 minutes. Take water breaks instead of coffee breaks.
8. Increase your drinking when you increase your mental activity level, your stress level, and your exercise level.
9. Drink the purest water available. Adding lemons to your water will help balance the pH in your body to make the water more purifying.
10. Perspire. Exercise to the point of perspiration or enjoy a steam bath. Sweat cleans the lymphatic system and bloodstream. It is one of the best detoxification avenues available to us. Do drink plenty of water afterwards to replace the loss of fluids. Drink more water in hot weather.

Choosing Quality Water for Health

There are many choices for water purification, but the underlying answer is that none of the choices are perfect. You, as the consumer, need to decide which one is best for you and your budget. Here are some keys to remember:

- Before using water, let cold taps run for a few minutes to flush out any lead that has leached into the water from the pipes.
- Use only the cold tap for drinking water and cooking, as there is a greater probability that the hot water contains lead, asbestos, and other pollutants from the hot water tank, if you have one.
- Use water filters to filter both your drinking water and your household supply.

- Avoid water gimmicks such as Vitaminwater. Here is the quote from the lawsuit of Center for Science in the Public Interest (CSPI) and Coca-Cola: "The marketing of vitaminwater will go down in history as one of the boldest and brashest attempts ever to affix a healthy halo to what is essentially a junk food, a non-carbonated soda," said CSPI executive director Michael F. Jacobson. "Vitaminwater, like Coca-Cola itself, promotes weight gain, obesity, diabetes, heart disease, and cannot deliver on any of the dishonest claims it has made over the years."

Bottled and Filtered Water: There is much controversy over quality water and the bottle industry. Plastic bottles, no matter what number, are polluting the land. The very best way to get quality water is to have a home filtration unit and use personal water glasses or high-quality bottles. This eliminates the guessing game as to which brand is the safest at the moment. And I do mean at the moment, because regulations in different cities and water quality change.

When traveling by car, I bring along a portable water purifier and personal water bottles to be refilled. This saves money and contributes less trash to the landfill.

Artesian water: is water from a well in which the water is brought to the surface by natural pressure or flow.

Ground water: comes from water underground in the water table, under pressure equal to or greater than atmospheric pressure, which does not come in contact with surface water. This must be pumped mechanically for bottling.

Mineral water: comes from an underground water source or spring that has been tapped at the spring opening or through a borehole. It has a constant level and proportion of minerals and trace elements at its source. No minerals may be added to this water.

Purified water: is bottled water that has been produced by distillation, deionization, reverse osmosis, or other processes and meets the legal definition so that it may be labeled as "purified" water or "demineralized" water.

Sparkling water: is water that has been carbonated. It can be a healthy alternative to soda and alcohol, but if it's loaded with fructose and other sweeteners, it may be no better than soda. Read the label! If the label says "naturally sparkling water," then the carbonation came from the same source as the water; but if it says "carbonated natural water," then the carbonation came from another source than the water. People suffering from intestinal disorders or ulcers should avoid carbonated water.

Spring water: comes from underground formations from which water flows naturally to the surface of the earth. Spring water must be collected only at the surface of the earth.

Tap water: is full of harmful chemicals that the body cannot use. It is known that pharmaceutical drugs—including antibiotics, hormones, painkillers, tranquilizers, and chemotherapy—and runoff from gardens and agricultural chemicals, such as fertilizers and pesticides, are detectable in much ground water, surface water, and tap water.

Steam-Distilled: this is one of the best. Distillation is the process of converting liquids into a vapor state by heating. The vapor cools and is condensed back into a liquid and stored. This method does remove all minerals and is sometimes called lifeless water. Some companies are selling minerals to add back into the water after the impurities have been removed. A high quality alfalfa supplement can add the minerals back into your diet easily.

Reverse Osmosis: This is one of the very best methods of producing quality water. A good source for reverse osmosis units for the home would include both predistillations and post distillations carbon filtrations for the highest level of quality and taste.

Here are some other tips for getting safe, pure water:

- For more information on safe water in your area, check out: www.epa/gov/safewater.
- Better choices of bottled water are Abita Spring, Evian, Ice Mountain, Glaceau Smart, Ozarks, Trinity Spring, Noah, Blue Star Sparkle, Arrowhead, Zephryhills, Mt. Valley Spring, Penta Water, Evamor, Jacobs Springs, and Nikken. Always read the labels to see if additives have been included.
- Before purchasing a water treatment unit, write, call, or visit the Web site "NSF International." This nonprofit testing and certification organization verifies manufacturers' claims and certifies that the materials used are nontoxic and structurally sound.

THE MIRACLE OF GREEN TEA

Tea has been an important beverage for thousands of years and has been a huge part of cultures in countries around the world, forming major parts of ceremonies and trade routes and even taking part in revolutions. But tea isn't just appreciated for its good taste and worldwide appeal; it also offers numerous health benefits.

Is any other food or drink reported to have as many health benefits as green tea? The Chinese have known about the medicinal benefits of green tea since ancient times, using it to treat everything from headaches to depression. In her book *Green Tea: The Natural Secret for a Healthier Life*, Nadine Taylor states that green tea has been used as a medicine in China for at least 4,000 years.

Today, scientific research in both Asia and the West provides hard evidence for the health benefits long associated with drinking green tea. There are numerous studies in the past and many just being released currently to exclaim the health benefits of green tea. To sum up, here are just a few medical conditions in which drinking green tea is reputed to be helpful:

- cancer
- rheumatoid arthritis
- high cholesterol levels
- cardiovascular disease
- infection
- impaired immune function

What makes green tea so special?

The secret of green tea lies in the fact that it is rich in catechin polyphenols, particularly epigallocatechin gallate (EGCG). EGCG is a powerful anti-oxidant. Besides inhibiting the growth of cancer cells, it kills cancer cells without harming healthy tissue. It has also been effective in lowering LDL cholesterol levels and inhibiting the abnormal formation of blood clots. The latter takes on added importance when you consider that blood clots are the leading cause of heart attacks and stroke. In a 1997 study, researchers from the University of Kansas determined that EGCG is twice as powerful as resveratrol.[6] Read more about this topic in this manual.

Why don't other teas have similar health-giving properties? Green, oolong, and black teas all come from the leaves of the Camellia sinensis plant. What sets green tea apart is the way it is processed. Green tea leaves are steamed, which prevents the EGCG compound from being oxidized. In contrast, black and oolong tea leaves are made from fermented leaves, which results in the EGCG being converted into other compounds that are not nearly as effective in preventing and fighting various diseases.

Harmful Effects?

To date, the only negative side effect reported from drinking green tea is insomnia due to the fact that it contains caffeine. However, green tea contains less caffeine than coffee: there are approximately thirty to sixty milligrams of caffeine in *six* eight ounce cups of tea, compared to over one hundred milligrams in just one eight ounce cup of coffee.

MILK, A NEW FOOD GROUP

Clean, raw milk from pastured cows is a complete and properly balanced food. You could live on it exclusively if you had to. Indeed, published accounts exist of people who have done just that[7]. What's in it that makes it so great? Let's look at the ingredients to see what makes it such a powerful food[8].

Proteins

Our bodies use amino acids as building blocks for protein. Depending on who you ask, we need twenty to twenty-two of them for this task. Nine of them are considered essential, in that we have to get them from our food. The remaining eleven to thirteen we can make from the first nine in the chemical factories of our bodies.

Raw cow's milk has all nine essential amino acids, saving our bodies the work of having to convert any into usable form. About 80% of the proteins in milk are caseins—reasonably heat stable but easy to digest. The remaining 20% or so fall into the class of whey proteins, many of which help with bodily processes.[9] Also easy to digest, but very heat-sensitive[10], these include key enzymes and enzyme inhibitors, antibodies, metal-binding proteins, vitamin-binding proteins, and several growth factors.[11]

Lactoferrin, an iron containing protein, has numerous beneficial properties, including improved absorption and assimilation of iron, anti-cancer properties, and anti-microbial action against several species of bacteria responsible for dental cavities[12]. Recent studies also reveal that it has powerful antiviral properties as well. This antiviral antibody provides resistance too many viruses, bacteria, and bacteria toxins and may help reduce the severity of asthma symptoms.[13]

It is important to note that studies have shown a significant loss of these important disease fighters when milk is heated in pasteurization.[14],[15]

Carbohydrates

Lactose, or milk sugar, is the primary carbohydrate in cow's milk. Made from one molecule each of the simple sugars glucose and galactose, it's known as a disaccharide. People with lactose intolerance, for one reason or another, no longer make the enzyme lactase and so can't digest milk sugar. This leads to some unsavory symptoms which, needless to say, the victims find rather unpleasant at best. Raw milk, with its lactose-digesting Lactobacilli bacteria intact, may allow people who traditionally have avoided milk to give it another try.

The end-result of lactose digestion is a substance called lactic acid (responsible for the sour taste in fermented dairy products). Lactic acid boosts the absorption of calcium, phosphorus and iron and has been shown to make milk proteins more digestible.[16]

Fats

Approximately two-thirds of the fat in milk is saturated. But is it good or bad for us? Saturated fats play a number of key roles in our bodies, from construction of cell membranes and key hormones to providing energy storage and padding for delicate organs, plus serving as a vehicle for important fat-soluble vitamins. More details will follow in this study, but the good news is that fats from foods God designed will not cause heart disease. Normal breast milk contains 50% fat. The fat in milk can cause our stomach lining to secrete a hormone (cholecystokinin or CCK) which, aside from boosting production and secretion of digestive enzymes, lets us know we've eaten enough.[17] With that trigger removed, non-fat dairy products and other fat-free foods can potentially help contribute to over-eating.

CLA, short for conjugated linoleic acid and abundant in milk from grass-fed cows, is a heavily-studied, polyunsaturated Omega-6 fatty acid with promising health benefits. Some of CLA's many potential benefits include: it raises metabolic rate, helps remove abdominal fat, boosts muscle growth, reduces resistance to insulin, strengthens the immune system, and lowers food allergy reactions. By design, raw milk from grass-fed cows has from three to five times more CLA than the amount found in the milk from feed lot cows.[18]

Vitamins

Volumes have been written about the two groups of vitamins, water and fat soluble, and their contribution to health. Whole raw milk has them both, and they're completely available for your body to use. Whether regulating your metabolism or helping the biochemical reactions that free energy from the food you eat, they're both present and ready to go to work for you.[19]

Minerals

Our bodies, each with biochemistry as unique as our fingerprints, are incredibly complex. Because of this, discussions of minerals, or of any nutrients for that matter, must deal with ranges rather than specific amounts.

Raw milk contains a broad selection of completely available minerals that range from the familiar calcium and phosphorus on down to trace elements, the functions of some, as yet, still rather unclear.

A sampling of the health benefits of calcium, an important element abundant in raw milk, includes but is not limited to: reduction in cancers, particularly of the colon; higher bone mineral density in people of every age; lower risk of osteoporosis and fractures in older adults; lowered risk of kidney stones; formation of strong teeth; and reduction of dental cavities. [20] [21]

An interesting feature of minerals as nutrients is the delicate balance they require with other minerals to function properly. For instance, calcium needs a proper ratio of two other macronutrients, phosphorus and magnesium, to be properly utilized by our bodies. Guess what? By design, all of the minerals in raw milk (from cows on properly maintained pasture) are in proper balance to one another, thus optimizing their benefit to us.[22]

Enzymes

The sixty plus (known) fully-intact and functional enzymes in raw milk have an amazing array of tasks to perform, each one of them essential in facilitating one key reaction or another.[23] Just keeping track of them would require a post-doctoral degree!

The most significant health benefit derived from food enzymes is the burden they take off our bodies. When we eat a food that contains enzymes devoted to its own digestion, it's that much less work for our pancreas. The enzymes found in raw milk break down starch, lactose (milk sugar), fat (triglycerides), and phosphate compounds, in that order, making milk more digestible and freeing up key minerals. Other enzymes help to protect milk from unwanted bacterial infection, making it safer for us to drink.[24]

Cholesterol

Milk contains about 3milligrams of cholesterol per gram—a decent amount. Our bodies make most of what we need, with that amount fluctuating based on what we get from our food. If we eat more, we make less. Either way, we need it. Why not let raw milk be one source?

Cholesterol is a protective/repair substance. A waxy plant steroid, our bodies uses it as a form of water-proofing and as a building block for a number of key hormones. It's natural, normal, and essential to our brains, liver, nerves, blood, bile—and indeed, every cell membrane.

Beneficial Bacteria

Through the process of fermentation, several strains of bacteria naturally present or added later (Lactobacillus, Leuconostoc, and Pediococcus, to name a few) can transform milk into an even more digestible food. [25]

Raw milk is a living food, a gift, with remarkable self-protective properties. But here's the twist: most foods tend to go south as they age (or spoil); raw milk just keeps getting better. Through helpful bacterial fermentation, you can expect an increase in enzymes, vitamins, mineral availability, and overall digestibility.[26] Not bad for old age!

What about Homogenization and pasteurization?

Pasteurization is heating food, in this case milk, to 161 degrees for fifteen seconds. This process denatures milk enzymes and changes its protein structure, making it difficult for our bodies to assimilate and digest. There's no debate about the effectiveness of pasteurization for killing unwanted bacteria. There's also no doubt that pasteurization gives dairy products a longer shelf life by lowering the presence of bacteria that cause spoilage. But pasteurization also kills desirable bacteria found in fresh milk, and it denatures milk enzymes that may be active in the human digestive tract when fresh milk is consumed.

Dr. Rex Russell, in his book *What the Bible Says About Healthy Living*, had this to say about pasteurization:

> Before it is pasteurized, whole milk contains many healthy proteins,
> enzymes, vitamins and minerals. A prime example is the vitamin folic

acid. A study reported that pasteurization denatures enzymes, decreasing the bioavailability of the folic acid and other nutrients found in raw milk. The heating in the process also destroys some of the vitamin and nutrients. The altered protein probable results in some people being allergic to dairy products. Calcium absorption is also decreased.[27]

Homogenization breaks up the larger butterfat globules in milk into very tiny globules which suspends them evenly in the milk. If milk is not homogenized, the fat globules are large enough to separate from the milk. An example of this is cream separating and rising to the top of a container. This means that the milk does not need stirring and may add to the storage life[28].

There are many theories regarding the study of homogenization in milk and the link to heart disease. The fact is the homogenization process began at the same time the climb in heart disease escalated but the connection is still vague. There are many on both sides of the aisle on this issue. Bottom line – milk has been consumed for over 5000 years but homogenization has only been on the rise in the last 70 years – around the same time our food has plummeted in nutrition and been modified at every corner to lengthen the time on the shelf and make our life simple.

So this means you will have to be the judge of whether or not to drink raw or store bought milk. I suggest reading up on this topic with an open mind. You may discover as I did that raw milk, the way God intended, is the best choice. For more reading and research I suggest reading the *Treasures of Healthy Living Bible Study* for an in-depth study.

GRAINS — GOODNESS AND FIBER

With the finest of wheat…

Deuteronomy 32:14

Whole Grains

WARM, FRESH BAKED bread is the true taste of the goodness of grains. Nothing compares to this satisfying taste and the health-promoting abilities of fresh whole wheat bread. If we want to eat the foods Jesus ate, then whole grains belong on the table.

When someone told me that I need to mill my own wheat and make my own bread, all I could picture was a horse walking around a stone mill in my backyard. My neighbors would definitely disagree with my choice. But fortunately, today we have the simple design of the Nutrimill to mill any grain, bean, or legume.

We have come far from the original design of bread. Today, the white flour used in over 99% of store purchased bread works the same as white sugar in the body. White flour has also been robbed of its color, taste, and smell. Twenty-six nutrients, plus the bran have been removed from wheat to produce white flour. Five of the removed nutrients are returned (in a chemical form) to produce "enriched" flour. What an enriching process!

Replacing white flour with freshly milled whole grain flours is a tremendous step in nutritional improvement. Freshly-milled flours have all of the natural oils and nutrients of the grain still intact. Once the grain is ground into flour by a flour mill, the flour can be placed in the refrigerator or freezer for up to one month before the natural oils go rancid. If the freshly-ground flour is left at room temperature, the natural oils will go rancid within forty-eight hours. After that time, the wheat germ, comprising ninety percent of the nutrients, is also rancid. "Rancid" basically means that the food item has spoiled and often will smell bad.

Eating rancid or spoiled food has obvious consequences, the least of which is increased toxicity to the body.

Invest in your health and make smart choices. Whole grains will add to your health, while processed, enriched, and fortified grains are imposters.

Journey through the field and tempt your taste with these grains of value:

Give us each day our daily bread.

Luke 11:3

Grains of Value

Amaranth: This poppy-seed sized grain, a botanical cousin to quinoa, has been a revered crop of the ancient Incas and Aztecs. It has a nutty and somewhat sweet flavor. It works best where a cohesive texture is desirable, as in spoon breads, casseroles, loaves, or hot cereals. Leftover cooked amaranth can be added in small quantities to muffins or quickie bread.

Barley: Barley is a short, stubby kernel with a hard outer shell. Pearled barley has the outer layer removed. Barley flour makes excellent pie crusts and cookies. It also mixes well with rice flour. It is the whitest of the whole grain flours and has a mild taste. It has no gluten and cannot be used with yeast.

Buckwheat: Buckwheat is not related to wheat and is in the grass family. Buckwheat groats are most often used as the basis for kasha. The flour is stronger flavored than many other flours and most often used in pancakes, waffles, and quick breads. A lighter colored and textured buckwheat flour can be made by placing hulled buckwheat groats in a blender and blending them into flour.

Cornmeal: Made from corn and popcorn, cornmeal is used primarily in cornbread, polenta, and mush. Only use organic corn due to the high percentage of GMO corn grown.

Kamut: A relative of durum of wheat, kamut is Egyptian wheat. Kamut can sometimes be used in place of wheat for those with wheat allergies. It produces excellent breads, pastas, and other baked goods. It has a light, slightly-buttery flavor and a golden color.

Millet: Millet was a staple food in many countries before the use of rice. Millet is the only grain that is not acid in the body and is highly recommended by most nutritionists. It has a high-quality protein and is rich in calcium, iron, and potassium. It is also very easy to digest. It is often used as a morning cereal or in soups, stews, casseroles, stuffing, and puddings. Millet flour tends to be heavy and bland in flavor. Oven temperatures should be reduced by twenty-five degrees for millet flour products.

Oats: Oats are an ideal cold-weather crop. They are second to amaranth and quinoa in protein, and rich in calcium, phosphorus, and iron. Since they have a slightly higher fat content, they produce a sense of warmness. Oat flour works well with cookies and in pie crusts.

Oat flour can be made by placing rolled or quick oats in the blender and blending until it is flour-like. Whole groats can be eaten uncooked for a chewy snack.

Quinoa: Traditionally grown in the Andes, the quinoa plant bears tan grains about the size of sesame seeds. Quinoa is similar to amaranth nutritionally; it yields a fluffier texture with a distinct flavor. Rinse quinoa well before cooking to remove its bitter coating. Quinoa flour has a stronger flavor and is best mixed with other flours. Quinoa is a great replacement for rice in your regular dishes. See the *Healthy Treasures Cookbook* for recipes that your family will enjoy.

Rice: Quickly becoming the most popular grain due to the rise in gluten intolerance, rice is mostly thought of in the varieties of white and brown. This is far from reality since rice comes in 18,000 different varieties and even brown rice comes in seven different bran colors such as: white, light brown, speckled brown, brown, red, variable purple and purple(black).

The design of rice is the same as wheat. It has the outer covering known as the bran which includes the nutrients of fiber, vitamin B, minerals and protein, the second part is the endosperm which includes the carbohydrates and more protein and vitamin B, then the germ which has the highest amount of vitamins, minerals and phytonutrients. With all these nutrients rice can move from the side dish to the main course. It is in itself a complete protein with all amino acids present.

Rice is sold as organic, whole grain and enriched. Ninety percent of rice sold in America is enriched and fortified with folate, iron, thiamin and niacin. No rice is currently enriched with vitamin A according to an interview with USARice.org.

Arsenic in rice has been the recent scare and is showing up in all varieties, even organic. Some growers such as Lundberg Rice Farms have seen the arsenic levels drop as they change farming practices. The FDA stated on September 6, 2013 that "Rice is an important staple for many people, and the arsenic levels that FDA found in the samples it evaluated were too low to cause any immediate or short-term adverse health effects." So as long as you trust the government then you have nothing to worry about. After interviewing Lundberg farms personally I would buy their rice as my first choice when available.

Rice and Rice Flour: Flour made from brown rice can be gritty in texture and taste, but it is excellent for thickening gravies and sauces. Baked products made only from rice flour tend to be crumbly. Brown rice flour works very well when mixed with barley flour.

Typical Varieties:

- Long-for winter, heartier, pilaf dishes. This variety will give you more flour for your dollar.
- Short/medium-for light, summer, creamier, sticky dishes. This variety will give you less flour.
- Basmati-for more winter dishes. Has a nutty flavor and produces strong-tasting flour.

*Any brown rice flour should be stored in the refrigerator because of the oil in the bran.

Spelt: Spelt is believed to be among the most ancient of cultivated wheats. It is higher in fiber and protein than wheat and is easily digested. Spelt is being promoted as a variety of wheat that is more tolerated by people with wheat and gluten sensitivities. It has a nutty aroma and flavor. The gluten content is more fragile than wheat, so it should be kneaded less in yeast recipes.

Storage

Whole grains should be kept in airtight containers in cool, dry places. They will last this way for a year or more. Adding a few bay leaves can help keep the grains bug free. If the grains are to be kept for a longer period of time, they should be kept in a five-gallon bucket with a "gamma-lid" for easy access. Five-gallon buckets can be purchased at local hardware stores, and gamma lids can be ordered from internet outlets. Some people have even acquired good icing containers from bakeries to use. These work perfectly for grains, beans, and other dry goods. Ask nicely and you may get one or more for free.

Cooking Suggestions

To dry roast, simply add the grain to an ungreased pan and place it over medium heat. Shake or stir the pan continuously for three to six minutes. Remove the pan from the heat before the grains turn too dark and start to burn.

When cooking grains, you may substitute chicken, beef, or vegetable stock for half or all of the water called for in the recipe. As a rule, I suggest replacing no more than half of the water with stock so that the delicate flavor of the grains is allowed to shine through. I also suggest that you use a low-sodium stock if you buy it canned—the full-strength commercial stocks are extremely salty.

Main Recipe for Grains (makes 3 cups)

This recipe works fine for quinoa, millet, barley, and coarse-grain bulgur. See chart below for cooking times.

1 cup quinoa, millet, barley, or coarse-grain bulgur
6 cups water
1 teaspoon kosher salt

Rinse grain in a colander. Bring the water and salt to a simmer. Add grain and reduce heat to a steady simmer. Cook for the times shown in the chart below. Pour into a sieve or fine colander and let drain for 10 minutes. Fluff with a fork and serve.

Cooking times for basic grains:

The cooking times below are to be used with the Main Recipe for Grains (above).
- Quinoa: 10 minutes
- Millet: 12 minutes
- Pearl barley: 45 minutes
- Coarse bulgur: 12 minutes, remove from heat, let sit for 5 minutes, then drain.

BARLEY

A land of wheat, and barley, of vines and fig trees, and pomegranates, a land of olive oil and honey.

Deuteronomy 8:8

The Bible is filled with references to barley, which is among the earliest known and most nourishing grains ever to be cultivated. In fact, the Feast of Unleavened Bread was an ancient barley harvest festival following the celebration of Passover.

Barley is a wonderful versatile cereal grain with a rich, nutlike flavor and an appealing, chewy, pasta-like consistency, the result of its gluten content. Its appearance resembles wheat berries, although it is slightly lighter in color. Sprouted barley is naturally high in maltose, a sugar that serves as the basis for both malt syrup sweetener and, when fermented, as an ingredient in beer and other alcoholic beverages.

Barley can be found in the market in various forms:

- **Hulled barley:** Like the name suggests, the outermost hull of the grain is all that gets removed. While this makes for a chewier grain that requires more soaking and cooking, it also makes for a more nutritious food. Hulled barley is also sometimes called "dehulled barley" or "un-pearled barley," and it is the one form of barley that would be considered whole grain.
- **Pearl barley:** Various degrees of polishing, or "pearling" take place in the production of pearl barley. In addition to a polishing off of the outermost hull, the grain's bran layer, and even parts of its inner endosperm layer, may be removed during the pearling process. In general, as you move from regular to medium to fine to baby pearl barley, you find an increasing loss of nutrients. Pearl barley is much less chewy and cooks more quickly than hulled barley, but it is also much lower in nutrients and would not be considered whole grain.
- **Pot/scotch barley:** In terms of processing, this form of barley falls in between hulled and pearl barley. It's been polished to remove its outer hull, but the polishing process is not continued for much longer so that a large amount of the remaining grain is left intact. While pot barley would not technically be considered whole grain,

and would lack some of the benefits of hulled barley, it is still a very reasonable nutritional choice and more nutrient-dense than pearl barley. In many countries, pot barley is popular in soups—thus the origin of its name.

- **Barley flakes:** Flattened and sliced, barley flakes are similar in shape to rolled oats. Barley flakes can be made from hulled, hulless, or pearl barley, and can vary significantly in nutrient content for this reason.
- **Barley grits:** Barley that has been toasted and cracked, barley grits are similar in appearance to bulgur. Barley grits can be made from hulled, hulless, or pearl barley, and can vary significantly in nutrient content for this reason.

Tips for Preparing Barley:

Like all grains, before cooking barley, rinse it thoroughly under running water and then remove any dirt or debris that you find. After rinsing, add one part barley to three and a half parts boiling water or broth. After the liquid has returned to a boil, turn down the heat, cover, and simmer. Pearled barley should be simmered for about one hour, while hulled barley should be cooked for about ninety minutes.

A Few Quick Serving Ideas:

- Mix barley flour with wheat flour to make breads and muffins that have a uniquely sweet and earthy taste.
- Use cracked barley or barley flakes to make hot cereal.
- Toss chilled, cooked hulled barley with chopped vegetables and dressing to make a tasty cold salad.
- Add barley to your favorite stews and soups to give them extra heartiness and flavor.
- Combine cooked barley and healthy sautéed mushrooms for a pilaf with an Eastern European twist.

Health Benefits:

- Helps with constipation
- Lowers cholesterol
- Heart disease prevention
- Lowers risk of type 2 diabetes
- Helps prevent gallstones
- Protects against childhood asthma (in a diet of fish and barley)
- Cancer prevention
- Helps with arthritis
- Development and repair of body tissue

Key Nutrients:

*B- vitamins	*Magnesium	* Protein
*Copper	*Phosphorus	* Vitamins A, C, D, E, K
*Fiber	*Selenium	* Omega 3

FACTS ABOUT FIBER

Earnestly desire the greater gifts, and I show you a still more excellent way.

1 Corinthians 12:31

It would be incomplete to study grains without understanding fiber and its role in your health. Did you know the following facts about fiber?

- Fiber decreases intestinal transit time, which moves food more quickly through the GI tract (less toxin build up).
- When you eat fiber, intestinal micro-flora benefit because of the more favorable medium in which they can live.
- An increased sense of fullness after eating fiber helps one eat less and enjoy it more.
- Increasing the daily intake of fiber by 10 grams decreases the risk of heart disease by 20 percent.
- By reducing fat intake and increasing fiber intake, one can reduce the risk of colon cancer by 30 percent.
- Fiber acts like an ambulance driver, as it takes dead Candida out of the body to the morgue (flushes it out).
- Fiber will give you more energy, help you control your weight, and really make a difference in your blood profile.

Definition:

Fiber is the structural material that makes up all plants. It is not a nutrient; therefore, it is not absorbed into the bloodstream. It is resistant to digestion by secretions of the digestive tract; therefore, it passes through the body. In this passing, it has some remarkable effects on our health.

Two Types of Fiber:

Insoluble Fiber: found in fruits and vegetables, wheat bran, whole grain cereals, whole wheat bread, nuts, and skins of fruits. Insoluble fiber:

- Plays an important role in bowel regularity.
- Absorbs and holds moisture, thereby producing larger stools and promoting regularity.

Soluble Fiber: found in fruits, nuts, legumes, plant seeds, and some vegetables (such as cabbage), and oat bran.

- Soluble fiber causes proper utilization of sugars and fats. It helps diabetics, hypoglycemia, insulin resistance, cholesterol issues, and high blood pressure.

*Good sources of both types of fiber are apples, wheat bran, whole grains, and dried fruits.

Practical Advice:
1. Eat the skins of organic potatoes, organic apples, and other fruits and vegetables.
2. Serve vegetables raw or steamed.
3. Use whole grain cereals, breads, and brown rice; avoid products made from white or highly-processed flour.
4. If you can't tolerate a particular high-fiber food, substitute something else. For example, replace beans with another vegetable.

How Much?
The National Cancer Institute recommends 25–30 grams of fiber per day. Others suggest 35–50 grams. Diabetics need over 50 grams daily. Research indicates that Americans eat approximately 8–12 grams of fiber per day. Increase fiber slowly in your diet.

Low Fiber Diets Lead To:
1) Constipation
2) High cholesterol
3) Cancer
4) Diverticulitis
5) Appendicitis—Appendicitis can occur when a hard lump of constipated stool blocks the opening of the appendix and bowel bacteria multiply in the appendix.
6) Hemorrhoids
7) Varicose Veins
8) Hiatal Hernia
9) Irritable Bowel Syndrome

10) Gallstones
11) Diabetes
12) Increase in Toxins in Bloodstream
13) Weight Gain and Obesity

Roles Fiber Plays:

1. Decreases likelihood of constipation. Fiber acts as a sponge, absorbing liquid, so that stools are softer and bulkier: therefore, they can pass through intestines more rapidly and easily.

2. Therefore, bowel disorders such as IBS, hemorrhoids, diverticulitis, cancer of the colon and rectum are reduced. In the US, 141,000 new cases of colon cancer are expected every year with 50,000 dying from this disease yearly. Do you want to be one of those statistics?

3. Lowers cholesterol and high blood pressure. Fiber latches onto the cholesterol in the bowel and prevents it from being reabsorbed into the bloodstream.

4. Researchers studied fiber intakes in twenty developed countries. Japan ranked the highest in fiber intake and had the lowest rank in coronary heart disease, while the US ranked the lowest in fiber intake and the highest in coronary heart disease. Soluble fiber, such as that found in oats, fruits, legumes, and different gums, is best for lowering cholesterol.

5. Decreases possibility of varicose veins, hiatal hernias, and gallstones.

6. Improves control of diabetes. Insulin needs are reduced.

7. Protection from toxic products.

8. Weight reduction and control.

9. Anti-carcinogenic. Wheat bran bonds nitrate (cancer-causing chemical), making it unavailable to form cancer-causing nitrosamines. Fiber, like chlorophyll, may prevent carcinogens from entering cells.

Fiber Mystery Unfolded

The appearance of the steel roller mill spelled the end of fiber consumption as we knew it. The roller mill, invented in 1870, was a quick and inexpensive way to separate the white inner substance (low in nutrients) of the grain from the outer bran and germ, both of which contain most of the key nutrients and nearly all of the fiber in the grain.

It was ideal for marketing. Whole wheat was a pain. The bugs ate the bran, and the germ would spoil. The inner white substance (endosperm) was resistant to spoilage (read "long shelf life"), and even the bugs ignored it, for the most part.

The popularity of refined products took off like a rocket. In many parts of America, in a very short time, cereal-fiber intake dropped by ninety percent. At the same time, consumption of fiber, including whole grains, beans, fresh vegetables, and fresh fruits, dropped (by fifty percent since 1910).

About this same time, sugar refining methods became more sophisticated, and sugar began to appear in our diets in large amounts. It is an excellent preservative and is added to most canned vegetables. In 1900, the average sugar consumption was 29 pounds per person per year. Now it is 140 pounds per person per year, with teenagers reaching even higher amounts.

As time has passed, more and more of the diet of western man has come to consist of sugar, fat, and white flour in various forms. Items such as ultra-refined breads, cereals, doughnuts, cakes, pies, cookies, instant potatoes, and white rice have become norms on American tables.

A Kernel of Truth

What has happened to the milling of wheat flour to make white flour is a good example of how we have been robbed of important nutrients that God created for our benefit. Some people refer to this as the "great grain robbery"!

When the wheat kernels are milled into white flour, the bran and the germ are removed. Only the endosperm remains in white flour. The chart on the following page shows how much nutrient value is lost.

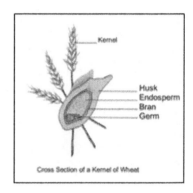

Cross Section of a Kernel of Wheat

Whole Wheat Flour Nutrients**	Nutrient Loss in White Flour*
Thiamine (B-1)	77%
*riboflavin (B-2)	67%
*niacin (B-3)	81%
pyridoxine (B-6)	72%
choline	30%
folic acid	67%
pantothenic acid	50%
vitamin E	86%
chromium	40%
manganese	86%
selenium	16%
zinc	98%
*iron	75%
cobalt	89%
calcium	60%
sodium	78%
potassium	77%
magnesium	85%
phosphorous	91%
molybdenum	48%
copper	68%
Fiber	89%

*Vitamins B-1, B-2, B-3, and iron are added to white flour in synthetic form by a process called "enrichment."

** Original source: Henry A. Schroeder, "Losses of Vitamins and Trace Minerals Resulting from Processing and Preservation of Foods," American Journal of Clinical Nutrition 241971); revalidated at www.ars.usda.gov/research/publications/publications.htm?seq.no_115=2-3150

A FIELD GUIDE TO FIBER

Remember: A healthy diet has 35-50 grams of fiber per day

FOOD	PORTION	SOLUBLE FIBER (g.)	INSOLUBLE FIBER (g.)	TOTAL FIBER (g.)
GRAINS				
Barley	¾ cup	1.8	2.7	4.5
Brown Rice	½ cup	0.2	1.6	1.8
Bulgur	½ cup	0.7	3.4	4.1
Rye Flour	2 ½ Tbsp	0.8	1.8	2.6
Rye Bread	1 slice			1.0
Whole Wheat	1 slice			1.6
Whole Wheat Spaghetti	½ cup	0.6	2.1	2.7
Wheat Germ	4 ½ Tbsp	1.0	4.2	5.2
Popcorn	2 cup			3.2
Oat Bran	1 cup	3.0	2.3	5.3
Oatmeal	1 cup	1.7	2.7	4.4
Millet	½ cup			1.8
Raisin Bran cereal	½ cup	1.0	12.0	13.8
LEGUMES				
Black Beans	½ cup	2.4	3.7	6.1
Butter Beans	½ cup	2.7	4.2	6.9
Kidney Beans	½ cup	2.8	4.1	6.9
Lentils	½ cup	0.6	4.6	5.2
Navy Beans	½ cup	2.2	4.3	6.5
Pinto Beans	½ cup	1.9	4.0	5.9
Split Peas	½ cup	1.1	2.0	3.1
VEGETABLES				
Artichoke	1 medium	2.2	4.3	6.5
Broccoli	½ cup	1.2	1.2	2.4
Brussels Sprouts	½ cup	2.0	1.8	3.8

FOOD	PORTION	SOLUBLE FIBER (g.)	INSOLUBLE FIBER (g.)	TOTAL FIBER (g.)
Carrots	½ cup	1.1	0.9	2.0
Sweet Potato	½ cup	1.8	2.3	4.1
Turnips	½ cup	1.7	3.1	4.8
Celery	½ cup	1.9	1.2	3.1
Corn	½ cup			3.9
Potato (Baked)	½ cup			3.8
Asparagus	½ cup			2.1
Green Beans	½ cup			2.1
Spinach	½ cup			2.0
FRUITS				
Apple	1 small	1.0	1.8	2.8
Avocado	½ cup	2.0	4.8	6.8
Blackberries	½ cup	0.7	1.8	2.5
Figs, dried	2	1.5	2.0	3.5
Guava	1	0.8	3.8	4.6
Kiwi	1	0.7	1.0	1.7
Mango	½	1.7	1.2	2.9
Prunes	½ cup	2.3	1.8	4.1
Raspberries	½ cup	0.5	1.1	1.6
Strawberries	¾ cup			2.0
Peach	1			1.6
Cantaloupe	¼ cup			1.4
Orange	1			1.2
Grapes	12			0.5
Raisins	2 Tbsp.			1.3
Banana	1			2.0
Grapefruit	½			1.7

BOUNTIFUL BEANS

Take wheat, barley, beans, lentils, millet, and spelt, put them into one vessel, and make them into bread for yourself.

Ezekiel 4:9

THIS RECIPE IN Ezekiel is for something that Bible scholars refer to as "Ezekiel's bread," which the prophet told the people to prepare during a siege of Jerusalem. It is one of the few specific recipes found in the Bible.

Neither Ezekiel nor the people who fixed and ate the bread knew it, but they were practicing a powerful healing technique that today's nutritionists call "augmentation." It simply means that a variety of grains used together packs much more potent food value and higher-quality protein than breads made from a single grain.

Health Benefits of Beans:

- Provide soluble fiber
- Lower harmful cholesterol
- Reduce blood pressure
- Keep blood sugar levels stabilized
- Stave off hunger
- Reduce the insulin requirements for people suffering diabetes
- Give energy
- Contain chemicals that inhibit the growth of cancer
- Help prevent and relieve constipation
- Stop hemorrhoids and other bowel-related problems from developing

Key Nutrients:

- Protein
- Vitamin C
- Fiber
- Iron
- Potassium
- Thiamine

As reported in 2 Samuel, beans were among the highly-nutritious foods sent to feed King David's hungry army and restore their strength:

…wheat, barley, flour, parched grain, beans, lentils, and parched seeds…for the people who were with him to eat; for they said, "The people are hungry and weary and thirsty in the wilderness."

2 Samuel 17: 28, 29

In these ancient times beans were often boiled with garlic, which produced a primitive version of a cough medicine that was said to stop even the most stubborn cough.

Now you don't have to eat beans morning, noon, and night to receive the benefits. A cup of cooked beans a day may be all that's needed, especially if your diet already includes similar foods that also fight cholesterol, cancer, and high blood pressure. Canned beans do not lose all their therapeutic strength as a result of processing but rinse them well to remove the salt and sugar in the sauce.

The health benefits make beans a great substitute for potatoes at the dinner table. You might even be able to improve the longevity of your marriage by serving your spouse one cup of beans every day.

One cup of beans contains:

- 17.9 grams of protein—the proteins in beans contain smaller quantities of protein then a steak, but the percentage of usable protein is over 50%.
- 6–7 grams of valuable fiber
- 12 grams of complex carbohydrates

Worried about the beans causing gas? That is easily remedied. When you increase bean consumption slowly, it gives your body a chance to adapt to the change in diet. You can also soak them overnight or flush them with boiling water, let them sit for about four hours, and then drain and cook in fresh water. Either method helps. Adding ginger to the soaking process will also help eliminate the gas. If your body still produces the embarrassing output, then consider adding enzyme supplements such as Beano or EZ Gest.

Adding Beans to Your Cooking

Beans are a great food, full of nutrition and add only 2–3% more fat to your diet. For those on a budget, beans will stretch your dollars and give your family a hearty, healthy meal. Learning to cook dry beans is easy to do with a little practice. Canned beans can be used also, but the cost is more. Also, you have to remember to rinse them well to avoid the added salt.

Using Beans in your Meal Planning:

Beans can be ground into flour and added to soups, casseroles, breads, etc. for a great protein pick up and more flavor. Start by substituting two tablespoons of your regular flour with bean flour. As you get used to the taste, then increase the amount. I did this in gravy, and it was very good and worked well as a thickener.

Common Varieties of Beans

Black Beans: small and black, but turn a dark brown when cooked. These can be used in soups and Mediterranean dishes. These are my favorite in refried beans, soup, and bean dip.

Black Eyed- Peas: small, oval-shaped, and creamy white, with a black spot on one side. These cook more quickly than most beans and reportedly cause less gas. Use these as a main dish or add them to a soup or salad.

Cranberry Beans: The speckled, cranberry-colored skin of these beans turns pink when cooked. Their flavor is nutty and similar to pinto beans. These taste great in chili, salads, soups, stews, and casseroles.

Fava Beans: a true Mediterranean treat. This large shaped bean is slightly bitter and goes well with pungent ingredients and zesty herbs.

Garbanzo Beans/Chick Peas: nut flavored and commonly pickled in vinegar and oil for salads. They can be served as a main dish or mashed and used as a binding agent in patties or meat loaves. A favorite cracker or vegetable dip from these beans is hummus.

Great Northern Beans: large, white beans used in soups, salads, casseroles, and baked bean dishes.

Kidney Beans: Large, red colored, and kidney shaped. They are popular for chili and salads.

Lima Beans: white, broad, and flat. They make an excellent main dish but also work well in soups and casseroles.

Lentils: an old world legume with a peppery taste. These beans are disc-shaped and about the size of a pea. They are the easiest and fastest to cook (30 minutes), since they require no advance soaking. Like soybeans, they are a complete protein and include all 8 essential amino acids. They can be served raw or cooked and used in making soups, casseroles, patties, and croquettes.

Navy Beans: named this because of their great use in the US Navy's dietary program. They are a version of Great Northern Beans. This flat, small, white bean is very versatile and can be used in any recipe calling for beans. It is the main ingredient in Boston Baked Beans.

Pinto Beans: same species as kidney beans and used in many Mexican dishes.

Split Peas: each variety has its own distinct flavor. They can be used for flour, as well as be put in soups, added to salads, and mashed for dips.

Soybeans: "King" of all beans when it comes to protein. Ounce for ounce, the soybean contains twice as much protein as meat, four times that of eggs, and twelve times that of milk. It is the only bean that is a complete protein, and it is loaded with vitamins.

Cooking Beans

Two options for cooking beans would be quick in the pressure cooker or slow in the crock pot. Cooking in the crock pot is done easily by placing one part beans, washed and cleaned, with three parts water in a crock pot. Cover and cook them on low overnight or for nine hours, until completely soft and tender. Once the beans are cooked they can be frozen in one or two cup measurements in the freezer in Ziploc bags. Label the bag with type of bean and date then lay it flat in the freezer for easy storage.

Bean Flour

Bean flours are a great way to add more nutrition to your cooking and baking. Flour can be made in your grain mill (Nutrimill) and then added to breads, casseroles, and even desserts without the soaking, boiling, and waiting you think you need with beans. Bean flours can be added in small quantities to any baked goods without a change in flavor or texture. If your family notices a flavor change, you can either cut back on the bean flour amount or add more, depending on how much they like the flavor. With the addition of bean flour, you can make your breads a complete source of protein.

NUTS AND SEEDS

I went down to the orchard of nut trees to see the blossoms of the valleys . . .

Song of Solomon 6:11

BOTANISTS TODAY BELIEVE that Solomon's "garden of nuts" referred to in this scripture was a rich grove of walnut trees. At the time, walnuts were prized for the oil they produced, which was regarded as only slightly inferior to olive oil, and for the valuable timber the trees provided. An added bonus is the fact that a walnut was a delicious treat and highly nutritious.

As the following verse from the book of Genesis shows, nuts were among the most treasured gifts one could offer: "Take some of the best products of the land in your bags, and carry down to the man as a present, a little balm, and a little honey, aromatic gum and myrrh, pistachio nuts and almonds." Genesis 43:11. Research shows that many people of that era owned olive or fig tree groves, but richer persons and kings also had almonds, walnuts and pistachios.

It is interesting to note the Israelites were not troubled by many of the health disorders that seem to plague us today, such as heart disease, cancer, and diabetes. This was in part because of the healthy nuts that were in their diet.

The tradition of nuts as a powerful healing food continues into the Middle Ages. Walnuts were considered so powerful that they were even included in a prescription to ward off the dreaded Black Plague that swept Europe during the Middle Ages.

Nuts have the right mixtures of natural ingredients, which have many benefits. They:

- Lower the risk of heart disease
- Help diabetes
- Lower total cholesterol
- Prevent Cancer

- Improves blood fluidity
- Increases arginine which reduces clots

The key nutrients in nuts are:

- Zinc
- Copper
- Iron
- Calcium
- Magnesium
- Phosphorous
- Polyphenols

All nuts seem to carry the same benefits. That includes just about any variety of nut you care to name—pistachios, peanuts, walnuts, almonds, Brazil nuts, cashews, acorns, chestnuts, or hazelnuts.

Nuts are just as much a part of the daily life and diet today in the countries surrounding the Mediterranean as they were in biblical times, when Jacob instructed Judah to send them as a gift to Joseph, governor of Egypt. That ancient tradition of giving nuts as offerings of peace and goodwill has been carried down through the centuries.

Foodie Facts: Substituting nuts for an equivalent amount of carbs reduces heart disease risk by 30%.

Substituting nuts for meat and dairy reduces heart disease risk by 45%.

Fat Content in Nuts and Seeds

Food—1 ounce	Fat (g)	Saturated Fat (g)
Almonds	15	1
Cashews, dry roasted	13	3
Chestnuts, roasted	1	0
Hazelnuts	18	1
Macadamia, roasted in oil	22	2
Peanuts, roasted in oil	14	2
Peanut Butter	16	3
Pistachios	14	2
Sesame Seeds	4	1
Sunflower seeds	14	2
Walnuts	16	2

All nuts contain high amounts of compounds called protease inhibitors, known to block cancer in test animals. Nuts are also rich in certain polyphenols, chemicals shown to thwart cancer in animals. However, while most nuts are generally healthy, peanuts are often contaminated by a mold called aflatoxin, which is a carcinogen.

Nut Varieties

FACTS	NUTRIENTS	FOOD OPTIONS
Almonds Cancer clinics recommend eating ten raw almonds.	High in potassium magnesium, protein, and phosphorous	Almond oil and almond butter are nutritious.
Cashews Grown primarily in India.	potassium, vitamin A, Magnesium, and fat	Don't consume large amounts. They contain high amounts of bad fat.
Chestnuts	Lowest fat content	Good raw, boiled, or roasted
Filbert or Hazelnuts Have a mild flavor.	potassium, sulfur, and calcium	Good cooked with vegetables and grains
Peanuts Often contaminated with aflatoxin (carcinogen) Member of hickory family	Complete protein and high fat content Potassium, vitamin A, essential fats	Raw, peanut butter Good for baking, candy, etc.
Pine Nuts Used in Middle Eastern and Italian dishes		Chewy and sweet. Good for salads or fruits
Pistachios May see holes in these Nuts made by a worm, which gives each nut its unique flavor.		Sweet, mild flavor

Walnuts

Oil is used in cooking	Potassium, magnesium, vitamin A, antioxidants	Good in all baking, salads, and desserts

It is best not to purchase roasted nuts or seeds because the oils become rancid when exposed to light and air. Consume only raw seeds and those tightly sealed in bags. Avoid nuts that are processed with added oil, sugar, or artificial flavors.

FLAXSEED

What is Flaxseed?

Flax is a blue flowering crop, with reddish or golden brown seeds that have been used since 650 B.C. for intestinal health. Research shows that flaxseeds can benefit bowel health, and protect against some cancers and heart disease.

Benefits of flaxseed

Flaxseed is a great source of soluble and insoluble fiber and essential fatty acids, also called omega-3 fatty acids. Moreover, it is a rich source of lignans, a type of phytoestrogen. Phytoestrogens are plant estrogens that can protect against certain types of cancer and control hot flashes during perimenopause.

Flax Fact:

Flaxseed has the highest concentration of Omega-3 fats in nature!

How is it eaten?

Flaxseeds are available in whole or ground form, also called flax meal. Ground flax (flax meal) is easily digestible, providing fiber for bowel regularity and beneficial Omega-3 fatty acids. Whole flaxseeds can be ground in a blender or coffee grinder. It is safe to bake with flax, but cooking at high temperatures can destroy beneficial oils. Whenever possible, add fresh ground flax meal after cooking. Everyone should have a minimum of 2 tablespoons of freshly ground flax seeds in their diet daily.

Learn More

To read the complete article about flaxseeds go to the Designed Healthy Living website. In summary, it is good for your head, your heart, your skin, your joints and much more…..

FANTASTIC FRUITS

And he will be like a tree firmly planted by streams of water, which yields its fruit in its season.

Psalm 1:3

Apricots

MANY BIBLE EXPERTS believe that the "apple" Adam and Eve ate in the Garden of Eden was probably an apricot and was simply misrepresented—mainly by painters in the Middle Ages. The Bible never mentions the apricot by name, but that doesn't meant it wasn't a major part of the healing of those times.

Several scholars state that the apricot, with the exception of the fig, is the most abundant fruit of the Holy Land. In Proverbs 25:11 (NASB), it is written, "Like apples of gold in settings of silver is a work spoken in right circumstances." In nearby Cyprus, apricots are known as "golden apples," which also is the literal translation of their Modern Greek name.

Health Benefits:
- Treat constipation
- Prevent Cancer
- Help with bowel disorder
- Benefit the skin, heart, muscles, and nerve tissues

Key Nutrients:
- Fiber
- Vitamin C
- Calcium/magnesium

- B-Complex
- Phosphorus
- Copper
- Fructose, glucose, and sucrose
- Manganese
- Iron
- Potassium
- Beta-carotene
- Lycopene
- Tannin
- Laetrile—this is derived from the pit and has been used to treat numerous disorders, including cancer. However, Laetrile contains enough cyanide to be fatal when eaten in large amounts, so I would suggest avoiding the pits.

Half a century ago, scientist G. S. Whipple, winner of the Nobel Prize, wrote that apricots were, "…equal to the liver in hemoglobin regeneration." In other words, they help clean the blood, which prevents us from aging before our time. Researchers point out that dried apricots may be even better for us than the raw fruit. Ten dried halves equal three raw apricots in beta-carotene content.

Apricots also may be effective in controlling high blood pressure and heading off premature heart attacks, as well as in boosting the critical levels of minerals that often decline in women after they reach menopause. That's because apricots contain large amounts of potassium (which scientists think is necessary in controlling blood pressure), calcium, copper, and iron.

In addition to all this, the good news about apricots is: A single apricot contains only 17 calories, a mere 0.4 grams of fat, and no cholesterol. It also contains vitamin A (2,768 international units of beta-carotene, or over half of the full day's recommended supply of 5,000 IU); vitamin C (11 milligrams or about 16 % of the RDA); some of the B vitamins; plus all that calcium, potassium, copper, and iron.

Grapes

Then they came to the valley of Eshcol, and from there cut down a branch with a single cluster of grapes. And they went carried on a pole between two men.

Numbers 13:23

That must have been some gigantic cluster of grapes! But such abundance was not unusual in the vineyards that were so important to the people of the Bible. Grapes were the first thing Noah planted after the Flood. As Genesis 9:20 says, "Now Noah started off as a farmer and proceeded to plant a vineyard."

In Bible times, grapes were eaten fresh, or dried and eaten as raisins, just as they are today. Most of the crop of the vineyards was made into juice, wine, and vinegar, although grapes were also pressed into cakes.

Nutrients included in grapes:
- Vitamins A, B, and C
- Minerals Boron, Zinc, and Potassium

Benefits of Grapes:
- Help protect against osteoporosis
- Fight tooth decay
- Stop viruses/Antiviral
- Antibacterial
- Anti-tumor agents
- Raise HDL (good cholesterol)

In years past, grapes were especially potent against the viruses like polio and herpes simplex. The reason, experts believe, is because grapes contain tannin, a virus fighter that is absorbed directly into the intestinal tract, where it does the most good.

Grapes have extraordinarily high levels of caffeic acid, which has been shown to be a strong anti-cancer substance. In pre-drugstore biblical days, grapes provided all of these health benefits. People didn't know what the grapes did, they just knew they were equally delicious eaten raw right off the vines, dried as raisins, boiled down into a sweet grape honey, or fermented into wine.

Resveratrol
> Thus says the Lord: "As the new wine is found in the cluster and one says, 'Do not destroy it, for a blessing is in it.'"
>
> Isaiah 65:8

For years researchers have advocated the benefits of drinking wine as a preventive measure against heart attacks. More recently, though, studies have determined that the alcohol content in red wine is not the factor responsible for reducing cardiovascular disease (CVD). Instead, researchers from all over the world are discovering that the antioxidants, called flavonoids, are the protective agents helping fight CVD and many other disease-related problems. And where can you find these helpful flavonoids? Purple grapes are the answer!

From the University of Florida, Patrick J. Bird, Ph. D. says, "Plants manufacture some 1,000 different flavonoids. But one—resveratrol—from the skin of the red grapes, seems to be most effective in the battle against heart disease. Resveratrol acts by decreasing the stickiness of blood cells that aid in clotting. Grapes are the richest source of resveratrol. Besides offering some protection against heart disease, it has been shown to decrease the activity of free-radical reactions that are linked to several cancers."[29]

Muscadine Grapes

Research has gone on to discover that resveratrol is not the only ingredient for promoting health found in the grape. Recent research has discovered that the Georgia-grown muscadine grape produces a unique phytochemcial, ellagic acid. Dr. Joseph Maroon, in his book *The Longevity Factor*, explains that this unique ellagic acid found in muscadine grapes is virtually absent in other grapes and has powerful antioxidant and anti-cancer properties. The polyphenols in muscadine grape skins have been shown to have positive effects in heart disease, high cholesterol, diabetes, metabolic syndrome, and other inflammatory conditions. In addition, one of the more interesting effects of the muscadine is its ability to repair the aging of DNA in our cells.[30]

Another scientist, Dr. Stephen G. Chaney, Professor at University North Carolina, had this to say in a personal interview: "Ellagic acid, found in the muscadine grape, blocks an enzyme that is involved in the formation of advanced glycation end products (AGE proteins), one of the central four mechanisms of cellular aging. (In layman's terms, AGE proteins are the sludge that builds up in our cells as we age) Resveratrol has no effect on this enzyme, but does block the other three key mechanisms of cellular aging." *Read more on Aging in this manual.

Summary of the most powerful grape of all: Muscadine

Health Effects:
- Powerful antioxidant
- Powerful antimicrobial properties
- Anticancer properties—to date, studied on breast, pancreas, esophagus, skin, colon, and prostate

Positive effects on:
- Heart disease
- High cholesterol
- Diabetes
- Metabolic syndrome
- Inflammation
- Inhibit AGE proteins

Figs

> For, lo, the winter is past, the rain is over and gone; the flowers appear on the earth; the time of singing of bird is come, and the voice of the turtle is heard in our land; the fig tree putted forth her green figs, and the vines with the tender grape give a good smell. Arise, my love, my fair one, and come away.
>
> Song of Solomon 2:11–13 KJV

Beginning with the Garden of Eden, the fig, with its astonishing health-giving and healing powers, is mentioned more than fifty times in the Bible. In fact, it is the first fruit specifically named in Genesis 3:7.

Figs, either fresh or dried, have been prized since ancient times for their sweetness and nutritional value. Greek and Roman athletes ate figs to increase their stamina and improve their performance. Even today in the Middle East, compote of dried fruits is a popular dessert. Dried figs, apricots and raisins are soaked overnight, boiled gently with a piece of cinnamon, and served cold with a sprinkling of orange or lemon juice.

Buying Figs

You can buy figs fresh, dried, or in tins. Fresh figs may range from golden yellow to deep purple-black. They should be fragrant and firm. Avoid those with soft spots or brown blotches, which mean the figs are old. Slightly shriveled skins indicate sweetness. Avoid figs that smell sour. Black mission figs are the most popular variety, but greenish-yellow-skinned Kadota and Calimyrna are also available. Dried or fresh, they keep best in the refrigerator. If you're buying dried figs, check what has been added. Some people are allergic to the sulfites often used to preserve dried figs and other dried fruits.

Benefits of Figs:

- Kill bacteria and roundworms
- Aid digestion
- Treat hemorrhoids
- Lower cholesterol
- Good for thymus gland
- Help immune system
- Useful in treating coughs, hoarseness, and respiratory and lung disorders
- Helpful with uterine fibroids
- Help build strong bones

Key Nutrients:
- Calcium   3–4 figs supply 100 milligrams
- Phosphorus
- Magnesium
- Potassium
- B vitamins
- Fiber
- Iron
- Vitamin C
- Vitamin E
- Phytochemicals

FRUITS AND HEALING

In the middle of its street, and on either side of the river was the tree of life bearing twelve kinds of fruit, yielding its fruit every month; and the leaves of the tree were for the healing of the nation.

Revelation 22:2

Here is a quick reference guide for many popular fruits and their healing potential:

Apples
- Contain 84% water; fiber; protein; minerals; carbohydrates; and vitamins A, B, and C
- Helps with:
    - Cleanse the bladder
    - Inflammation of colon
    - Intestinal infections
    - Diarrhea
    - Arthritis
    - Acid stomach
    - Lower blood cholesterol
    - Lower blood pressure
    - Herpes and viruses
    - Protect against danger from radiation therapy and x-rays
    - Stabilize blood sugar

Here's a tip: To ripen fruits faster, leave them in a plastic or paper bag. The bag traps the ethylene gas that is produced by the fruit and acts as a ripening agent. Apples give off a large amount of gas, so you can speed ripening by placing an apple in the bag with other fruits.

Avocado
- Contains high amounts of good fats. Great for the hypoglycemic.
- Helps with:
- Fatigue
    - Hypoglycemia
    - Urinary infections
    - Nerves

Bananas
- Excellent for infants and children. Great amount of potassium and Vitamin C
- Helps with:Nerves
    - Hypertension
    - Hemorrhoids
    - Heart Disorders
    - Ulcers
    - Diarrhea
    - High Blood Pressure
    - Edema
    - Intestinal disturbances
    - Muscle contraction and relaxation
    - Supply good bacteria in colon

Blueberry
- High in Vitamin C, potassium, fiber, manganese. The blue pigment may be a powerful liver protector.
- Helps with:
    - Hypoglycemia
    - Tinnitus (ringing in ears)
    - Rejuvenates pancreas

Blackberry
- All berries are high in fiber.
- Helps with:

- Chronic appendicitis
    - Constipation
    - Diarrhea
    - Build blood
    - Anemia

Cherries
- Prevent tooth decay by stopping plaque formation with black cherry juice.
- Cherries remove toxins from the body and aid in gallbladder and liver function.
- Helps with:
    - Gout (excellent for this)
    - Rheumatism
    - Paralysis
    - Arthritis
    - Stunted growth
    - Obesity

Cranberry
- Wonderful for bladder infections. High in Vitamin C
- Helps with:
    - Kidneys and Bladder
    - Asthma
    - Skin
    - Intestinal antiseptic

Figs
- Fig juice is wonderful for destroying intestinal parasites.
- Provide high amounts of fiber
- Kill bacteria
- Destroy roundworms
- Help hemorrhoids
- Anti-cancer agent
- Aid digestion

Grapes

- Full of antioxidants
- Stimulate the liver
- Increase energy
- Helps with:
  - Skin
  - Fever
  - Constipation
  - Cancer
  - Edema
  - Heart Palpitation
  - Remove toxins and cleanse all tissues and glands

Grapefruit

- The whole fruit, pectin, pulp, and fibrous parts are important.
- Good for a healthy heart
- High in potassium and Vitamin C
- Helps with:
  - Cardiovascular system
  - Chest congestion
  - Protect the arteries
  - Cancer protection
  - Lower blood cholesterol

Lemons and Pineapple

- Wonderful liver stimulants and solvents for uric acid and other toxins.
- Fresh pineapple contains manganese, which is essential for certain digestive enzymes, so it is a wonderful digestive aid.
- Cleanses bloodstream and liver
- Helps with:
  - Inflammation
  - Colds, influenza, and sore throat
  - Bronchitis
  - Asthma
  - Digestion
  - Heartburn

- Diabetes
- Scurvy
- Rheumatism
- Fevers

Melons
- Rich in Vitamin C, Beta Carotene

Oranges
- Contain high amounts of Vitamin C and A.
- Choose oranges that do not look like they are a wax imitation. Oranges that are picked green before the acid can turn to fructose (natural fruit sugar) cause a problem for most people. They are sprayed orange to look appealing. Choose those that do not look perfect.
- Helps with:
    - Anti-cancer
    - Sinus, allergies
    - All upper respiratory
    - Collagen formation
    - Colds, flu symptoms
    - Gum disease
    - Bruising

Papaya
- Breaks down unwanted substances, including uric and toxic acids in body.
- Great to add to infant formula to help digestion.
- Helps with:
    - Acidosis
    - Colon disorders
    - Enzymes
    - Digestion
    - Ulcers

Peaches
- Contain beta-carotene, potassium, and fiber
- Prevent cancer and heart disease
- Helps with colon disorders

Pears
- Have a very high insoluble fiber
- Natural laxative
- Helps with:
    - Arthritis
    - Gout
    - Lungs and stomach

Pomegranate
- Helps:
    - Diarrhea
    - Sore throat and fever

Prunes
- A prune is a dried plum.
- The benzoic acid present in plums is used for liver disease, blood poisoning, and kidney disorders.
- High fiber content is found in prunes, but not in the juice.
- Helps:
    - Lower blood cholesterol
    - Constipation
    - Prevent parasites

Raspberry
- Liver tonic
- Diarrhea remedy
- Helps with:
    - Frequent urination
    - Impotence

Strawberries
- Strawberries contain high amounts of Vitamin C, potassium, and have lots of fiber.
- Great antioxidants, strawberries can block the transformations of nitrosamine, a powerful cancer-causing substance.
- The viruses that strawberries can destroy in the body are retro-viruses and herpes viruses.

- Protect against:
  - Viruses and cancer
  - DNA damage
  - Herpes simplex virus, skin disorders, and acne

Here is a tip: Do not remove the strawberry caps until you are ready to eat, to keep the Vitamin C intact. To understand this idea better, think about what happens when you slice an apple. The oxidation is obvious since it begins to yellow. The same is true of the strawberry; removing its cap allows it to start oxidation. Better yet – keep the cap on and throw the whole strawberry into the blender. The cap is nutritious.

Watermelon
- Natural diuretic
- Blood purifier
- Cleanses tissues
- Helps canker sores in mouth

VICTORIOUS
VEGETABLES

Every green plant for food…

Genesis 1:30

E VERYTHING THAT GROWS out of the ground contains proteins, especially our vegetables. Contrary to past beliefs, vegetarians can receive all the needed proteins from vegetables. Combining two or three per meal will assure sufficient protein intake. Vegetables also contain the needed essential fatty acids, vitamins, minerals, trace minerals, and many unidentified nutrients.

Cruciferous Vegetables—The Magnificent Twelve

Preventing disease is a must for all of us and eating more vegetables will make that happen. But not all vegetables are alike. These twelve magnificent vegetables (vegetable families) are the power fighters against cancer and heart disease, the two top killers in our country. Flowers found on these vegetable plants have four petals that botanical historians describe as resembling the crucifix or cross, thus they are called "cruciferous."

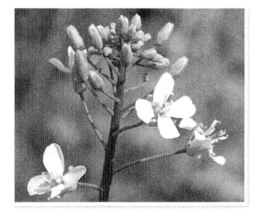

Dr. Couey's latest research shows that the phytochemicals in the cruciferous vegetables are repairing DNA in the cell. Repairing DNA means making a mutated cell into a healthy cell. Isn't that just how Jesus dying on the cross also covers and repairs our sin and removes it! Praise the Lord – that is a Praise Tickle in the finest!

It is best to consume three, one cup servings

from this list *every* day. Eat one cup raw and two cups slightly steamed, except for horseradish. Use horseradish grated fresh in sauces and spreads. Alternate the vegetables daily.

If consuming cruciferous vegetables gives you an upset stomach or causes bloating or gas, you may lack alpha-glactosidase, an enzyme that breaks down certain complex sugars. Add these vegetables gradually so that your system can tolerate them. Start with half a cup two times a week and increase. There are enzyme supplements to assist people who need help with digesting these foods.

The Magnificent Twelve:

1. Broccoli
2. Brussels Sprouts
3. Cabbage
4. Cauliflower
5. Horseradish
6. Kale
7. Kohlrabi
8. Mustard Greens
9. Radishes
10. Rutabaga
11. Turnip
12. Watercress

Scientists are discovering that the phytochemicals, many known and unknown natural chemicals, in our foods are more important than the vitamins and minerals they contain!

Following is a short breakdown of these twelve vegetables and their benefits and nutrients. This is just a brief look and not at all conclusive.

Broccoli
Health Benefits:
- Lowers the risk of cancer, primarily of the rectum, colon, esophagus, larynx, lung, prostate, oral cavity, pharynx, and stomach
- Protects against heart disease, cataracts, constipation and hemorrhoids, diabetes, arthritis, and allergies
- Helps normalize body fluid levels
- Controls high blood pressure
- Promotes bowel health

Key Nutrients:
- 26 phytonutrients and still counting and discovering
- Beta-carotene
- Chromium
- Fiber
- Calcium
- Copper
- Iron

- Magnesium
- Phosphorus
- Sodium
- Vitamin B
- Zinc

- Manganese
- Potassium
- Sodium
- Vitamin C

It is believed that green vegetables, along with dark orange vegetables, act as antidotes to the cancer process that continues for years after exposure to carcinogens. Always buy green broccoli to ensure freshness. Never buy it when it is yellow. Steam broccoli lightly to keeps its nutrients intact. Wash broccoli under cold running water. Remove the leaves, if any, and add them to fresh salads. You can also peel and slice the stalks and add them to stir-fry dishes and vegetable dips.

Brussels Sprouts
Health Benefits:
- Inhibit cancer
- Protect against estrogen-related cancer
- Inhibit the formation of polyps
- Detoxify aflatoxin, a fungal mold linked to cancer, particularly liver cancer. Aflatoxin often contaminates peanuts, corn, and rice.

A juice made of Brussels sprouts, string beans, lettuce, and carrots provides the needed elements to regenerate and improve the insulin-producing capacity of the pancreas.

Key Nutrients:
- 17 phytochemicals and counting
- Beta-carotene
- Copper
- Iron
- Manganese
- Potassium
- Vitamin B
- Vitamin E
- Zinc

- Amino Acids
- Calcium
- Fiber
- Magnesium
- Phosphorus
- Sodium
- Vitamin C
- Vitamin K

Brussels Sprouts should be firm with compact, bright green heads. The stems should be white with no worm holes. They should be stored unwashed, untrimmed, and in a perforated plastic bag for up to five days in the refrigerator. Remove any wilted or yellowed leaves before storing.

Soak sprouts in a basin of warm water for ten minutes, then rinse with cool water. Remove the coarse outer leaves and trim the ends. To ensure even cooking, cut a small x into the bottom of the stem. Cook sprouts just until tender.

Cabbage

Health Benefits:

- Kills bacteria and viruses
- Prevents cancer, particularly of colon
- Prevents and heals ulcers
- The juice stimulates the immune system

Key Nutrients:

- 21 phytochemicals and counting
- Calcium
- Iron
- Manganese
- Potassium
- Vitamin B
- Vitamin E
- Zinc
- Beta-carotene
- Fiber
- Magnesium
- Phosphorus
- Sodium
- Vitamin C
- Vitamin K

For generations cabbage has been known for its therapeutic effect in conditions of scurvy, diseases of the eyes, gout, rheumatism, pyorrhea, asthma, tuberculosis, cancer, and gangrene. Within cabbages are chemicals called indoles that block cancer formation. Also, there are dithiolthiones, which suppress the activation of cancer-causing (carcinogenic) substances. These include: chlorophyll, certain flavonoids, isothiocyanates, phenols (like caffeic), ferulic, acetic acid, and vitamins E and C.

The healing factors in cabbage are present only when taken raw, usually as a juice. The best cabbage to use is fresh spring and summer cabbage. Fall cabbage is less effective, and winter cabbage is the least effective. To make a suitable drink, add three quarters cabbage juice to one quarter celery juice. Celery also contains an anti-ulcer factor. For extra flavor, add pineapple juice to the cabbage juice. Drink a quart a day if you're suffering from any ulcer. Within three weeks, if not less, you should feel some results. The sulfur content helps fight infection and protects the skin from eczema and other rashes.

Different types of cabbages to consume include Napa (Chinese cabbage), bok choy, and celery cabbage. All are from the cruciferous family and contain anti-cancer chemicals. A number of studies have determined that raw cabbage and Cole slaw give protection against stomach cancer.

Cauliflower

Health Benefits:

- Reduces risk of cancer—Cauliflower contains compounds, like indoles, which stimulate the natural defenses to neutralize carcinogens.
- Slows tumor growth
- Lowers circulating estrogen levels in the body
- Neutralize carcinogens

Key Nutrients:

- 13 phytochemicals and counting
- Calcium
- Iron
- Phosphorus
- Vitamins C, B, and K
- Beta-carotene
- Fiber
- Magnesium
- Potassium

Look for cauliflower heads that are firm, with compact florets. Not yellowed.

Horseradish

Health Benefits:

- Anti-cancer properties
- Blood sugar balancing action
- Diuretic
- Expectorant
- Good for digestion

Key Nutrients:

- Calcium
- Fiber
- Iron
- Magnesium
- Potassium
- Vitamins C and B

Kale

Kale is notes as one of the best cancer-fighting vegetables we have on our planet. Unfortunately, due to its coarse texture and strong flavor, we do not usually have it in our diets. Kale is the richest of all leafy greens in carotenoids, powerful anti-cancer agents. All leafy greens lead the list of cancer preventatives.

Health Benefits:
- Best cancer fighting vegetable
- Good for arthritis
- Helps with osteoporosis
- Protects smokers against lung cancer

Key Nutrients:
- Vitamins A, B, and C
- Calcium and magnesium
- Iron, sulfur, sodium, potassium, phosphorous, and chlorophyll

Heat destroys some of the carotenoids, but the resulting balance is more available to the body, and the chlorophyll content does not seem to be affected. It is wise to consume kale both in the raw and cooked forms. The taste is mild so it works well in smoothies and soups.

Kohlrabi

Health Benefits or Improves:
- Diabetes
- Fresh juice has been used in China to stop nosebleeds
- Improves eyesight
- Indigestion
- Jaundice
- Lymph system and alcoholism
- Reduces the effects of cigarette smoking
- Reduces the risk of hormone-dependent cancers

This vegetable contains high amounts of vitamin C, calcium, and potassium. It is also a good source of fiber. The taste is like a mild turnip. Try it raw or cooked.

Mustard Greens

Health Benefits:
- Inhibits tumor growth
- Protects against cancer and heart disease
- Strengthen the immune system
- Contain high amounts of calcium, iron, vitamin A, and niacin.
- Superior to spinach, because of the lower oxalic acid content, so the benefit of the calcium is not lost.

Key Nutrients:
- 10 phytochemicals and counting
- Calcium/Magnesium
- Iron
- potassium
- Vitamins B, C, K, and E
- Beta-carotene
- Fiber
- Phosphorus
- Sodium
- zinc

Radishes

Health Benefits:
- Cleanse gallbladder and liver
- Diuretic
- Good for colds and flu
- Help respiratory infections
- Remove mucus
- Soothe headaches and heal laryngitis
- Stimulate the appetite

The key nutrients are very similar to all the other cruciferous vegetables listed on this worksheet. They can be eaten raw, cooked, or pickled.

Rutabaga

Health Benefits:
- Clears up mucus and congestion
- Has an alkalizing effect on the body
- Contains anti-cancer qualities
- High fiber

- Nutrient dense – high energy

Note: The most nutritious root plants include: carrots, parsnips, turnips, celery roots, radishes, onions, garlic, daikon, ginger, horseradish, and rutabagas.

Turnips
Health Benefits:
- Balance the calcium in the body
- Being a cruciferous vegetable, they have cancer-fighting compounds
- Help asthma and bronchitis
- Reduce mucus
- Relieve sore throats

Key Nutrients:
- High amounts of antioxidants, mainly vitamins A and C
- High in calcium, iron, and niacin

Turnips are good raw or shredded for salads. Cook the green tops like any other green or steam lightly or add to soups and stews.

Researchers theorize that antioxidants, particularly vitamin C and carotenoids, like beta-carotene in fruits and vegetables, retard oxidation damage to the lens of the eye. Oxidation is primarily responsible for age-related cataract formation.

Watercress
Watercress is another member of the mustard family, and is the last of the Magnificent Twelve.

Health Benefits—good for:
- Anemia
- Appetite stimulation
- Arthritis and emotional problems
- Blood purification
- Calcium deficiencies
- Cataract conditions
- Liver and pancreas problems
- Thyroid problems

Key Nutrients:
- High in potassium, sulfur, vitamin A, calcium, and iron
- Copper
- Magnesium
- Sodium
- Potassium
- Iodine

The Brazilians have used syrup from watercress as a remedy for tuberculosis. Anyone who is ill should chew on a few stalks of watercress daily. You can also add it to juices and chop it fresh for salads. It is excellent when added to bulgur wheat salads.

The Bottom Line

Vegetables contain many cancer fighting substances: *Indoles* (cancer inhibitors) are found in cabbage and related vegetables like broccoli, Brussels sprouts, cauliflower, kale, and mustard greens—all members of the Magnificent Twelve. *Sterols* are found in cucumbers, terpines, and citrus fruits. *Polyacetylenes* are in parsley; *sulfur compounds* in garlic; and *osoflavones* in peanuts, beans, and peas. *Lignin's* come from flaxseeds, *quinones* from rosemary, and *triterpenoids* from licorice roots.

Obese people and heavy alcohol drinkers have a far greater incidence of cancer when their diet is lacking fresh vegetables and fruits. There are many other reports, confirming our contention, that whole, fresh vegetable and fruits were designed by the Creator of all things to nourish and protect us. You can be truly blessed with good health by regularly consuming the Magnificent Twelve and other vegetables.

Pesticides and Fertilizers

All plant life has natural built-in protection against insects. These "protective pesticides" are usually in micro amounts and safe for human consumption. How amazing, the vegetable kingdom has their "defense system" too.

According to Sharon Hornick, Ph.D., a USDA researcher, chemical fertilizers adversely affect the quality of crops. In addition to nutritional losses, chemically fertilized crops have decreases in the following areas: taste, storage ability, insect resistance, and disease resistance. Chemically grown kale, for example, was found to have only one-half the vitamin C content of organically-grown kale.

Going Green

Before cleaners were vying for the title of "going green," there were the original greens—leafy greens. Lettuces contain a rich source of vitamins A, B, C, zinc, calcium, and potassium. There are dozens of varieties of lettuce, but only a few are grown commercially. This means you can experiment with various new flavors in your own garden. Here are some ideas.

Arugula: This unique peppery-flavored lettuce is a perfect accent to pasta and salads.

Beet greens: These are best used in juices. The leafy tops of beets are rich in carotenes and minerals. The tops should be crisp and dark green in color.

Bibb: This lettuce looks like a miniature romaine, and its flavor is outstanding.

Boston or Butter leaf lettuce: has a soft buttery flavor and texture.

Endive: Looks like leaf lettuce but is more tolerant to cold. Its flavor is sharp and almost peppery.

Green leaf: is a beautiful green, curly leaf variety that really stands out in a salad mixture. The flavor can sometimes seem a little flat.

Iceberg: This lettuce is the most popular but far from the tastiest.

Red Leaf: This curly, dark auburn-red colored leaf has a soft texture and a mild sweet taste.

Romaine: This is a head lettuce, although the leaves do not close together in a round ball—rather they are long and flat.

Spinach: is a nutritious bonanza. It prevents cells form undergoing mutation, reduces the risk of cancers, and blocks the formation of nitrosamines.

When shopping for lettuce, freshness is of key importance. Never choose lettuce that has wilted or yellowed leaves. Another way to inspect it is to look at the base; it should always be hard with a pale white or pinkish color.

PROTECTIVE FOODS FOR HEART HEALTH AND CANCER PREVENTION

RESEARCH REVEALS THAT certain food groups can reduce the risk of heart disease, cancer, diabetes, and allergies. These foods contain protective nutrients, such as high levels of antioxidants, vitamin C, vitamin E, beta-carotene, and zinc. They also contain properties, such as phytochemicals in plants, which contribute to their color, aroma, and flavor. These foods provide a composite of elements that work together; therefore, it's always best to eat the whole food close to God's design. Refer to the Produce Shopping Guide on the website for guidelines on purchasing organic verses non-organic produce.

Foods high in Omega-3: flax seeds, flax seed oil, salmon, mackerel, haddock, rainbow trout, sardines, tuna, halibut, and bluefish

Foods high in soluble fiber: oats, oat bran, organic soybeans, barley, carrots, garbanzo beans, apples, citrus fruits, bananas, melons, broccoli, potatoes, dried peas, and beans

Fruits high in vitamin C and pectin: organic apples, pears, black currants, citrus fruits, strawberries, red currants, goose berries, tomatoes, raspberries, and blackberries

Fruits high in vitamin C and bioflavonoids: lemons, limes, oranges, grapefruit, tomatoes, pumpkins, potatoes, strawberries, and green and red peppers

Foods containing plant sterols: eggplant, cabbage, organic soybeans, peanuts, brown rice, barley, sweet potatoes, and avocados

High Potassium Foods: potatoes, avocadoes, orange juice, raisins, sweet potatoes, tomatoes, squash, bananas, dried apricots, flounder, and salmon

Foods high in monounsaturated fats: avocadoes, almonds, pecans, cashews, hazelnuts, and olive oil

Oils high in essential fatty acids: flax seed oil, sunflower oil, safflower oil, organic soybean oil, and whole grains

Foods high in vitamin E: whole grains, wheat germ, organic soybeans, nuts, seeds, and fresh veggies

Foods high in sulfur compounds and allium: onions, garlic, leeks, chives, and scallions

Foods high in magnesium: green veggies, figs, lemons, grapefruit, apples, organic soybeans, almonds, nuts, seeds, and wheat.

Foods high in B vitamins: whole grains, eggs and leafy greens

Foods high in zinc: whole grains, eggs, and pumpkin seeds

Foods high in calcium: organic low fat or nonfat yogurt and almonds

Veggies high in carotenoids: dark greens, carrots, red peppers, apricots, peaches, yellow squash, and sweet potatoes

Veggies containing indoles and isothiocynates: cruciferous veggies (see complete listing under this heading in this book)

Veggies high in chlorophyll: parsley and dark leafy greens such as spinach, kale, collard greens, mustard greens, and turnip greens

Foods Associated with Specific Cancer Sites[31]

Bladder Cancer	Fruits and Vegetables, adequate water
Breast Cancer	Olive oil, physical activity
Cervical Cancer	Folic Acid, Fruits and Vegetables
Colorectal Cancer	Vegetables, especially cruciferous vegetables, calcium, Vitamin D, Whole Wheat bran, physical activity
Kidney Cancer	Fruits and vegetables, especially orange and dark green colors
Mouth, Throat, and Esophagus Cancer	Fruits and Vegetables
Liver Cancer	Vegetables, especially yellow and green ones
Lung Cancer	Fruit and Vegetables
Ovarian Cancer	Vegetables, especially green ones
Pancreatic Cancer	Fruits and vegetables, especially green and yellow ones
Prostate Cancer	Possibly cooked tomatoes, soybeans, flaxseed and adequate selenium intake (with Vitamin E)
Stomach Cancer	Fresh fruits and vegetables, especially tomatoes

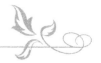

HERBS AND SPICES

For the earth is the Lord's and all it contains.

1 Corinthians 10:26

ARE HERBS THE secret to life? Who knows if herbs are the answer to longevity, but with all the coverage they have received throughout history, it appears that many believe it. Herbs themselves have been one of God's special blessings. They have provided people with flavors, fragrances, and medicinal benefits. New aromatic herbs may fill your home with pleasing scents while changing the most ordinary food into a memorable meal.

The words "herbs" and "spices" can be used interchangeably. Their medicinal and culinary value is equal. "Herbs" refers to all parts of the plant—roots, stems, leaves, flowers, seeds, essential oils, bark, and fruit.

Herbs must be used with a light touch. To alter the flavor of any basic dish, you can prepare it with different combinations of herbs or spices. Listed below are some of the common varieties of herbs that you can grow and harvest or buy at your local store. The health benefits are listed also so that you can see God's treasures in these wonderful plants.

Dried vs. Fresh: While dried herbs are convenient, they don't generally have the same purity of flavor as fresh herbs. To make sure the herbs are still fresh, check if they are green and not faded. Crush a few leaves to see if the aroma is still strong. Always store them in an air-tight container away from light and heat. Use three times more herbs if substituting fresh for dried.

Allspice: A berry used whole, ground, or pressed with the leaves for their oil. The flavor is a blend of cinnamon, cloves, and nutmeg. Allspice has anti-inflammatory, antioxidant, and anticancer properties.

Anise: Anise has a licorice flavor. It is used in baked goods, oriental dishes, soups, and cakes. This spice has been used for treating digestive problems, coughs, bronchitis, and asthma.

Basil: Sweet, warm flavor with an aromatic odor. Use whole or ground. It relieves a variety of digestive problems, including stomach cramps, vomiting, and constipation.

Bay Leaves: Pungent flavor. Use whole leaf but remove before serving. Bay leaves are an aid to relaxation and help to manage stress. These are also good for migraines and diabetes.

Caraway: Spicy taste and aromatic smell. Caraway helps soothe stomach disorders and aid digestion.

Cayenne: Flavors hot, spicy dishes, eggs, and beans. Good for chronic pain, such as arthritis. Cayenne can relive pain when allied on the skin.

Celery Seed: Strong taste, which resembles the vegetable. Celery seed assists the flow of urine through the kidneys, aids the digestive system, and helps to relieve the symptoms of arthritis and rheumatism.

Chives: Sweet, mild flavor like that of an onion. Chives stimulate the appetite, ease digestion, and help relieve gas.

Cilantro: Use it fresh; excellent in salads, fish, chicken, rice, beans, and Mexican dishes.

Cinnamon: Sweet, pungent flavor. Cinnamon has antiseptic properties and can be used as a digestive aid to relieve nausea, vomiting, diarrhea, and indigestion.

Coriander: (Also called cilantro.) Light lemon, orangey flavor. It is available whole or ground. Coriander helps relieve indigestion, gas, and diarrhea.

Cumin: has a strong smell and is bitterly hot. Cumin helps to relieve gas, aid digestion, and treat colic and headaches. It is also an antioxidant. Use seeds sparingly.

Dill: has a pungent aroma. Dill is used as a digestive aid, is good for the kidneys and spleen, lowers blood pressure, improves poor appetite, and increases circulation. It also helps milk production in nursing mothers.

Fennel: Sweet, hot flavor. Both seeds and leaves are used. Fennel has a gentle laxative effect, relieves infant colic, and helps both to stimulate the onset of menstruation and to promote milk production in nursing mothers.

Ginger: A pungent root, this aromatic spice is sold fresh, dried, or ground. Ginger has been used for nausea, morning sickness, upset stomach, indigestion, vomiting, motion sickness, and cramps.

Mace: Mace is the outer covering of nutmeg. Mace is a bit more delicate in flavor than nutmeg, but they can be used interchangeably. See Nutmeg for health benefits.

Marjoram: May be used dried or green. This is effective as a digestive aid, reduces fevers, and relieves cold and flu symptoms.

Mint: has a sweet, cool aftertaste. Mint is useful in easing insomnia, upset stomachs, and nervous tension. It is also good for digestion.

Nutmeg: Whole or ground, it has a sweet and spicy flavor. Nutmeg aids in relieving pain, abdominal swelling, indigestion, and diarrhea.

Oregano: Aromatic, slightly bitter. Oregano helps treat fever, vomiting, diarrhea, and skin problems.

Paprika: Pungent and peppery, but not hot. The phytosterols in paprika have anticancer, anti-inflammatory, and immune-boosting properties.

Parsley: Mild flavor. Best when used fresh, but can be used dried. Good for indigestion, measles, lungs, and spleen.

Rosemary: Very aromatic; can be used fresh or dried. Rosemary stimulates the appetite, aids digestion and circulation, helps prevent food poisoning, and relieves spasms in irritable bowel syndrome.

Sage: Aromatic, slightly bitter. Good for canker sores, bleeding gums, sore throat, lungs, diabetes, and wounds. Sage is also an antioxidant.

Savory: This herb blends well with other herbs to make a salt-free seasoning that is good for stews, vegetable dishes, pizza toppings, roasting meats, and fish. By itself it adds flavor to bean dishes and evens helps with the digestion of beans.

Tarragon: Pungent, hot taste. This is an appetite stimulant, eases digestion and toothache pain, and stimulates urine flow. It also expels intestinal parasites.

Thyme: (Also lemon thyme.) Warm, slightly pungent flavor. Thyme has been used as a digestive aid, cough and laryngitis remedy, and antiseptic. Use thyme butter over vegetables.

Turmeric: Musky, slightly bitter, and peppery taste. Turmeric is anti-inflammatory and antibacterial. It also reduces cholesterol levels and improves blood vessel health.

Vanilla: Sweet and rich taste. The vanilla bean has been used to invigorate and strengthen the body and promote healing. It can also be used to relieve gas and treat abnormal menstruation. Only use natural extract in cooking, not imitation.

SALT

You are the salt of the earth; but if the salt has become tasteless, how will it be made salty again?
Matthew 5:13

Salt has been around since the earth was formed, and even today it is known for its own unique flavor that can change a bland recipe into a pleasing favorite. But salt is used for so much more.

Salt has at least three unique qualities:

1. *A little salt sets the flavor in food.*
2. *Salt is a preservative.* Our grandparents used salt to cure food to be used later. Ham, beef jerky, and salted fish were staples of their diets.

3. *Salt has healing properties.* It kills most germs on contact. It burns when it hits a raw spot, but is very effective in cleansing a wound so that it can heal. "Don't rub salt in my wounds," is a statement often heard when a person is hurt from good advice.

Facts about salt:

- Refined salts, even in saltwater concentration, will kill saltwater fish. So, what do you think is the fate of our internal organs when fed commercial salt?
- 100 pounds of water from the Dead Sea yields 24 pounds of salt. Whereas, 100 pounds of water from the Atlantic Ocean yields 6 pounds of salt.
- Fruits and vegetables are nearly salt-free. This means that a vegetarian diet will eventually create an anemic condition and other salt-starvation diseases. That is why many vegetarians crave salty snack foods. Only when salt is added to fruits and vegetables can saliva and gastric secretions readily break down carbohydrates.
- Human salt consumption accounts for only 7% of the total salt production; the balance (93%) is used by the chemical industry and in manufacturing for things like manufacturing explosives, chlorine gas, agro-fertilizers, and in the plastics industry.
- Magnesium is extracted out of common table salt. Because the chemical industry needs pure sodium and chloride, vital magnesium is taken out to make the salt flow more smoothly, which means it can be sold for a better profit on the chemical market.
- Flowing agents are added to salt. To prevent moisture from being reabsorbed, salt refiners also add alumino-silicate of sodium or yellow prussiate of soda as desiccants, plus bleaches. This salt is then sold in stores for human consumption. The problem is that this alteration makes the salt unable to combine with human body fluids, so it causes health disturbances.
- Ocean salt alone possesses the power to restore wholeness to the human internal seas, our bodies' fluids.
- Every one of the body's 92 essential minerals is found in the ocean.
- Salt refining: When most salts are harvested, they are put through a series of harsh steps that cracks the molecular structure, robs its essential minerals, and adulterates the salt with chemical additives to make it free-flowing. It is then bleached and iodized. This refining process makes the salt poisonous to your body because it takes out the essential nutrients and aliveness present in sun-cured sea salt.
- Celtic sea salt is the lowest in sodium and the richest in precious beneficial elements of all the salts available.
- Once re-dissolved in water or in the moisture of food as it cooks, Celtic Sea Salt bears an amazing likeness to human blood and body fluids.[32]

Hold the Salt Shaker

Salt is forty percent sodium and sixty percent chloride, and both of these nutrients are essential in our diet. But salt is even more essential for the processed food industry. Adding salt to processed foods constitutes an "eat more" strategy all its own; it makes food taste better because it heightens flavors, reduces bitterness, and enhances sweetness. Salt is perfect for processed foods. It is cheap. It keeps foods from becoming discolored, and it extends shelf life. Even better, it binds water and makes food weigh more so that you pay more for heavier packages.

Foods made from scratch, with real ingredients in their original forms, are relatively low in salt. But only about ten percent of the salt in the American diet comes from salt added at the table. The other ninety percent is already added in processed foods, where it cannot be avoided unless you cook your meals using whole foods.[33]

Foods with a high amount of sodium added include, but are not limited to: bouillon cubes; canned meats, vegetables, and beans; peanut butter; salad dressings; luncheon meats; meat tenderizers; packaged spice mixes; potato chips; corn chips; pretzels; processed cheeses; crackers; and salted nuts.[34]

Most of today's salt is mined and comes from large deposits left by dried salt lakes believed to be left from a great worldwide flood. (Don't you love those facts?) Here is a breakdown of the different types of salt available on the market:

- **Table salt** is refined, fine grain salts with additives that make it free flowing.
- **Iodized salt** is table salt with iodine added to it.
- **Kosher salt** is an additive-free, coarse-grained salt. It is used by some Jews and cooks to help remove blood from meat.
- **Sea salt** is the result of evaporation of sea water. It is also mined in the dried beds from the flood era, as mentioned above. Sea salt doesn't contain iodine or any other additives. However, if you use sea salt, you typically don't have to worry about not getting enough iodine in your diet because iodine is available in many other foods, including dairy products, seafood, and many processed foods. If you favor foods with fewer additives, you may prefer sea salt.
- **Celtic salt** is natural, solar evaporated sea salt that's been hand harvested from the Atlantic marshes in France. It has a mellow, sweet-salty flavor.
- **Rock salt** has a grayish cast because it is not refined, which means it retains more of its minerals. It comes in chunky crystals and is predominantly used in making ice cream and in snow and ice removal.
- **Seasoned salt** is table salt combined with other flavoring ingredients, examples being onion salt, garlic salt, and celery salt.
- **Salt substitutes** are products containing little or no sodium. Typically these are chemically based.[35]

VINEGAR

Almost as old as the universe itself vinegar is one of the oldest condiments in the world. It is believed to have been discovered quite by accident. Wine was exposed to air and, voila, "sour wine" or vinegar was invented. Too tart to drink, too precious to throw away, creative experimentation proved that soured wine had fascinating properties—one of them being the power to pickle!

Ancient Egyptians and Chinese used vinegar thousands of years before Christ, and its use is mentioned in both the Old and New Testaments. Traces of vinegar were discovered in an Egyptian vessel dating back 5,000 years.

Babylonians used it for cleaning and preserving food. And in Rome, legionnaires drank vinegar before battle, believing it gave them strength and courage. After the fighting was over, vinegar was applied as a disinfectant to cleanse wounds inflicted by swords.

Today, vinegar—specifically apple cider vinegar—is touted as being a miracle cure. Whether that is true or false is your decision. One way to find out is to take the apple cider vinegar test: mix 1–2 teaspoons of organic apple cider vinegar with raw honey or agave nectar (to sweeten) in an 8 ounce glass of distilled water. Drink it first thing in the morning and one hour before lunch and dinner. Continue this for one month. This tonic may cause the following results:

- Combat mucus
- Fight kidney and bladder problems
- Help prevent constipation
- Improve digestion
- Relieve chronic fatigue
- Relieve headaches
- Rid the body of toxins
- Strengthen the heart

Dr. Carol Johnston, professor at Arizona State University, just released a study proving that apple cider vinegar taken at bedtime favorably affects waking blood sugar in type 2 diabetics and helps reduce glucose levels by up to six percent.[36] Johnston also discovered that her subjects were losing weight.

These are just a few examples of the issues that can be alleviated with apple cider vinegar (ACV). Organic ACV comes as a brownish liquid with a cobweb substance known as the "mother" in the bottle. This is the highest quality of vinegar available. This treasure delivers enzymes, potassium, phosphorus, magnesium, iron, copper, trace minerals, essential amino acids, and many other powerful nutrients. Be aware that clear white vinegar has been refined and bleached. Some white vinegar is even processed from coal tar!

Tips for Using Vinegars

- Light, Bright Salads—you can cut down or eliminate oil by simply tossing greens with a shake of organic, store-bought or homemade herbal vinegar.
- Guilt-Free Desserts—In Italy it is common practice to dip fresh strawberries into a little bowl of balsamic vinegar before eating. This is truly a must-try treat. Unlike traditional chocolate or caramel dunks, balsamic vinegar actually draws out and enhances flavor rather than masking it. Try sticking other fruits like banana slices, apple wedges, and peach or pear slices on toothpicks and dipping them in balsamic vinegar for exciting variety.
- Thirst Quencher—Stir a tablespoon of apple cider or fruit vinegar into iced water for a tantalizing thirst quencher. This is said to regulate body temperature and clear up bad complexion.
- Diva Dip—Cider, balsamic, or herbal vinegars poured into the dip bowl make a delightfully light substitute for sour cream, mayonnaise, and other fatty dips. You can dunk veggies until your heart's content.
- Balsamic Dip for Bread—Here's a super quick and delicious Old World dish from Italy. Combine 1/2 cup balsamic vinegar, 3 tablespoons extra virgin olive oil, 5 cloves of roasted mashed garlic, and 1 teaspoon of freshly-grated black pepper into a jar. Shake well and let draw in fridge until flavors meld. Serve with chunks of crusty bread for dipping. This is an elegant appetizer, easy picnic dish, or good impromptu supper.
- Getting the Most out of Soup Stocks—Adding a squirt of white wine or apple cider vinegar (about 2 tablespoons per pound of bones) to the stock pot helps leach valuable calcium from the bones. You will gain calcium and the sour taste will be gone.
- Potassium-Rich Tea—If your stamina needs improving, you may need more potassium in your diet. One teaspoon full of cider vinegar per cup of herbal tea can fill the bill. Also, a dash in place of lemon perks up tea.

Making Your Own

Herb Vinegar: Gather a few sprigs of fresh garden herbs—the more you use the stronger it will be. You can use basil, dill, rosemary, sage, tarragon, thyme, mint, chives, or whatever is handy in your herb patch. Wash, pat dry, and put the herbs in a sterilized bottle. Cover them with apple cider, malt, or any wine vinegar or blend of vinegars you desire. Let draw for two weeks, then strain and bottle. Peeled garlic cloves, shallots, peppercorns, chilies, juniper berries, or other spices and seasonings can also be added.

Fruit Vinegar: Use raspberries, cranberries, blueberries, or your choice of fruit in place of herbs. Create unique flavors by adding orange peel, lemon zest, pomegranate seeds, nutmeg pod, cinnamon stick, or other sweet things to the bottle. For the best in fruit infused vinegar, use white wine or champagne vinegar. Let draw for two weeks, then strain and bottle.

Purchasing and Storing Vinegars

Vinegars are used in cooking and baking, for making salad dressings, to transform milk into a buttermilk substitute, and in marinades. But which type of vinegar should you use?[37] Here is a quick breakdown of the types you can purchase in the store:

- **Balsamic vinegar** is the most expensive because it is aged for a longer period of time. The longer it's aged, the sweeter and thicker it gets, and the more expensive too.
- **Red and white wine vinegars** are more "everyday" vinegars. They are good for salad dressings and marinades. Red wine vinegar is best used with heartier flavors and foods, like beef and vegetables. White wine vinegar is best for chicken and fish dishes.
- **Apple cider vinegar** is mild and inexpensive, and it works well in salad dressings. Since it is mild, it's a good choice for marinating fish or chicken. It's also good for making flavored vinegars.
- **Rice vinegar** is the mildest of all, with much less acidity than other vinegars. It's often used in Asian or Chinese cooking.
- **Plain distilled vinegar** is made from grain alcohol and has a very sharp, unpleasant taste.

Lemon and lime juices can be substituted for red wine, white wine, apple cider, and rice wine vinegars. Don't use them in place of balsamic vinegar, because you won't get the same depth of flavor.

All vinegars should be stored tightly closed in a cool, dark place. They will last for about a year after opening. After that time, the flavors will diminish. Purchase expensive vinegars in very small quantities, and be sure to use them within one year.

FACTS ABOUT FATS

WHEN IT COMES to fat, we have the good, the bad, the ugly and the confusing. But how do you know one from the other?

Fats are a concentrated source for energy as well as building blocks for cell membranes and hormones. Do you remember those fat soluble vitamins—A, D, E, and K? These vitamins need fat from your diet as their "Amtrak" to move them to the body's tissues. Consuming a low-fat or no-fat diet increases the risk of a deficiency of vitamins A, D, E, and K in your cells. These vitamins bypass the blood stream and go directly into the lymph system to help build your immune system. The blood stream is water-based, so it cannot transport these fat soluble nutrients.

Here are some fat facts:

Good Fats
- Highest caloric density, above protein and carbohydrates, 9 calories per gram
- One tablespoon contains 120 calories.
- Act as an intestinal lubricant
- Keep you feeling full longer and satisfied after a meal by staying in the digestive tract longer
- Generate body heat
- Soothe the nerves and protect the nerve cells
- Required by all body cells

Bad Fats or too much of the Good
- Excess fat is stored in the liver, arteries around the heart, and in all tissues
- High fat consumption is linked to cancer, obesity, and heart disease
- Fat cells in the body can grow to 1000 times their size to store more fat

- Some fats are created within the body and others are required from our food consumption. Those required from food are known as *essential*.

Fats in Everyday Foods

There are four basic types of dietary fats: mono-unsaturated, polyunsaturated, saturated, and trans-fats.

Saturated Fatty Acids

These fats are usually considered the "bad" fats but some experts will disagree. They come primarily from animal and dairy products and recognized as being hard at room temperature. These fats replace good fats in the body's cellular structure when there is a deficiency of good fats in the diet. A high intake of these fats is believed to increase cholesterol, heart disease, and cancer. Foods with saturated fat considered bad include: bacon, beef, hard cheese, milk, and pork. Fatty meat products also have a high percentage of saturated fats. Saturated fats considered good include organic or raw butter, coconut oil and palm oil. However, foods such as animal and dairy products farmed in organic ways have proven to be a healthier option than the medicated meats and dairy products. This has lead to the confusion of bad verses good fats.

Saturated fatty acids can also be produced in our body by eating refined sugars. Saturated fatty acids are not essential to our diet and contribute to obesity and health problems. Saturated fatty acids produced by eating refined sugars interfere with essential fatty acid functions in the body and increase the chances of a fatty liver disease.

Monounsaturated and Polyunsaturated Fatty Acids

Poly and Mono are close relatives and are the good guys. These fats remain liquid at room temperature. Good sources of monounsaturated fat include: olive oil; almond, peanut, pistachio, pecan, organic canola oil; and foods such as avocados, nuts, and seeds (including flax seeds). Olive oil, organic canola oil, and some nuts also contain important polyunsaturated fat. ***Caution:*** canola oil has been found to high amounts of trans fats in it, so I would avoid if possible.

Polyunsaturated fatty acids

The polyunsaturated fatty acid family includes GLA (see article in this book), Linoleic acid and alpha-linolenic acid (ALA), Omega 3 and omega 6.

Omega-3

This is an essential fatty acid also known as alpha-linolenic acid (ALA). In addition to ALA, there are two other Omega-3 fatty acids—docosahexanoic acid (DHA) and eicosapentaenoic acid (EPA).

Benefits associated with Omega-3, include:

- Helps with all forms of arthritis
- Helps control viral infections
- Reduces cholesterol and triglycerides levels
- Lowers the risk of heart attack, stroke, and hardening of the arteries
- Improves psoriasis
- Improves immune response
- Lowers effect of harmful body chemicals
- Improves brain function
- Reduces severity of migraine headaches
- Improves liver and pancreas function
- Reduces cystic fibrosis

Good sources of Omega-3 include pumpkin seed oil, flax seeds, walnuts, pine nuts, pecans, cold water fish (sardines, mackerel, and salmon), wheat germ, sesame seed oil, organic corn oil, safflower, organic soy bean, and sunflower oils.

Omega - 6

Omega-6 fatty acids are also essential fatty acids.

Benefits associated with Omega 6

- Brain function
- Normal growth and development
- Stimulate hair and skin growth
- Maintain bone health
- Regulate metabolism
- Maintain the reproductive system
- Helps with diabetic neuropathy, rheumatoid arthritis, allergies, ADHD, breast cancer. Hypertension, eczema, MS and PMS

A healthy diet contains a balance of omega-3 and omega-6 fatty acids. Omega-3 fatty acids help reduce inflammation, and some omega-6 fatty acids tend to promote inflammation. The typical American diet tends to contain 14 - 25 times more omega-6 fatty acids than omega-3 fatty acids.

Following the Three Principles, which is similar to the proven Mediterranean diet, has a healthy balance between omega-3 and omega-6 fatty acids. Many studies have shown that people who follow this diet are less likely to develop heart disease. The Mediterranean diet does not include much meat (which is high in omega-6 fatty acids, though grass fed beef has a more favorable omega-3 to omega-6 fatty acid ratio) and emphasizes foods rich in omega-3 fatty acids, including whole grains, fresh fruits and vegetables, fish, olive oil, garlic, as well as moderate wine consumption.

For complete understanding of fats in the body and how they create inflammation view the DVD series that accompanies this study; *Treasures of Healthy Living* DVD with Dr. Couey – Inflammation.

Trans Fatty Acids

Trans fatty acids are formed when natural vegetable oil is heated and hydrogenated to converted the liquid into a solid. Man's attempt to improve on God's design continues to fail. Although it prolongs the shelf life of popular foods it also destroys the beneficial essential fatty acids.

Hydrogenated oils, such as margarine, fats that are industrially hardened to avoid rancidity, and processed foods, such as pies, cakes, and potato chips, are other major sources of trans fatty acids.

Hints to Follow when Using Oils

- Purchase cold or expeller-pressed oils (unrefined).
- Avoid hardened oils (hydrogenated or partially hydrogenated).
- Never re-use oil that has been used for frying.
- All oils should be stored in a cool, dark cupboard.
- Never consume oil that smells rancid.
- Olive oil maintains a longer shelf life than most oils.
- Don't let oils heat to smoking.
- To sauté or stir fry, use 2 tablespoons of water in the oil.
- Take one vitamin E capsule (must be a natural supplement and not synthetic), puncture it (small hole), and put the capsule in the bottle of olive oil. This will keep the oil from going rancid.

Olives and Olive Oil—the Favored Fat

The Lord called your name, a green olive tree, beautiful in fruit and form.

Jeremiah 11:16

The olive was certainly one of the most valuable and versatile trees of biblical times. It is mentioned over 140 times throughout the Bible. Since the time of Noah, the olive branch has been seen as a symbol of peace. For the Jews, olive oil was a sign of God's blessing, because it represents all that is best in life. It has been noted that no tree is more closely associated with the history of man and the development of civilization than the olive.

Olives and olive oil have been studied extensively to prove their healing properties. They:

- Strengthen cell membranes.
- Retard cancer growth.
- Lower bad cholesterol and raise good cholesterol.
- Reduce the production of gallstones.
- Have healing and anti-inflammatory effects.
- Stimulate bile flow.
- Improve brain maturation.
- Stimulate the production of fat-digesting enzymes in the pancreas.
- Reduce gastric acidity.
- Protect against ulcers.
- Help prevent constipation.
- Aid normal bone growth.
- Are rich in vitamin E, one of the best antioxidants available.

Olive oil is most suitable for both expectant and nursing mothers because it encourages development of the infant's nervous system before and after birth.

If you're trying to reduce the amount of fat in your diet to avoid the risk of heart attack, think of olive oil as an ideal replacement for other oils and fats. Anything you can sauté in butter, you can sauté in olive oil. Not only will you be helping your heart, but also you will be pleasing your taste buds.

Defining the highest quality oil:

- Virgin—physical (not chemical) extraction at a specific temp. This oil has no deterioration or defects in the olives and has a free acidity not more than 2%.
- Extra Virgin—free acidity not more than 0.8%, no defects in olives
- Olive Oil (not labeled Virgin or Extra Virgin) is a blend of refined and virgin oil. It has a free acidity not more than 1%

TIP: It may cost a little more, but extra virgin olive oil contains more of those natural ingredients credited with fighting heart disease. The purer the oil, the more your heart will love you. When it comes to olive oil, you get what you pay for. This is one area that you need to invest in and buy the higher quality. Remember, food is cheaper than medicine.

- Refined—defects found in base oil are removed and blended with other refined oils. Refined with charcoal and chemical/physical filters
- Cold pressed—first pressing with hydraulic press and temp less than 27˚ C
- Cold extraction—oil separated and filtered by percolation or centrifuge
- Estate grown—95% of the oil must come from a single estate.
- Blended—oil is from different estates.
- Light and extra light—refined (chemically/physically) for lighter color, fragrance, and taste

Things to look for on the label:
- Country of origin – better to have one country/ location that various sources
- When it was bottled – we want the freshest quality
- Use by date
- Once opened use in 60–90 days

Tips for using your high-quality olive oil:
- Use olive oil in a spritz bottle in lieu of cooking spray.
- Freeze or refrigerate olive oil to use as a spread.
- Store olive oil in dark glass, stainless steel, or tin.
- Store olive oil in a cool, dark place.

Olive Oil Folk Remedies

1. *For shiny hair:* After shampooing, rub in a mixture of olive oil and egg yolk and the juice of one lemon. Leave in for 5 minutes and wash out.
2. *To prevent dandruff:* Rub a mixture of olive oil and cologne into the hair and scalp. Rinse.
3. *For dry skin:* Make a face mask with an avocado and olive oil. Leave on for 10 minutes and rinse.
4. *To prevent wrinkles:* Rub a mixture of olive oil and the juice of a lemon into the skin before going to bed.
5. *To soften the skin:* Mix together equal parts of olive oil and salt. Massage in well, and then wash off with cool water.
6. *For weak nails:* Soak the nails for 5 minutes in warm olive oil. Then pat the nails with white iodine.
7. *For tired feet:* Massage with olive oil.
8. *For aching muscles:* Massage with a mixture of olive oil and rosemary.

9. *To clear acne*: Try a mixture of 8 ounces of olive oil and 10 drops of lavender oil.
10. *To remove oil from fabric*: rub baking soda in and let sit overnight. Then wash.
11. *For pregnancy and baby care*: Helps with gas in babies. Heals cradle cap, dry skin, and diaper rash. Mix water and oil to soothe sore nipples.
12. *For Pet Health*: 1 TBS on food for shiny hair, less shedding, and hairballs. Heals raw skin that is licked and foot pads. Removes ticks and ear mites.

YOGURT

YOGURT IS NOT mentioned by name in the Bible, but tradition says that an angel promised Abraham that he would live a long life if he ate the biblical version of yogurt. He lived to be 175 years old! Today, in parts of the Middle East, Southeastern Europe, and much of Asia, yogurt is a staple food and has been enjoyed for thousands of years.

Yogurt is highly regarded for many reasons. It:

- Has bone-building calcium.
- Prevents colds.
- Prevents allergic reactions.
- Helps fight cancer—specifically colon and breast.
- Strengthens the body's immune system.
- Lowers bad cholesterol levels.
- Prevents dangerous intestinal infections.
- Improves bowel function.
- Prevents gas and bloating.
- Blocks ulcers.
- Is a natural antibiotic—research has pinpointed at least seven different antibiotics—while helping to restore the good bacteria needed for proper digestion and assimilation of nutrients.
- Destroys E. coli and Salmonella.
- Contains Tryptophan, which can act as a mild sedative; but for some reason, the tryptophan/yogurt combination perks you up rather than slows you down. That's why a cup of yogurt in the afternoon may be a better pick-me-up snack than the jolt of caffeine from a cup of coffee.

In addition, yogurt is a great source of:

- Protein.
- Calcium.
- Potassium.
- Vitamin B, especially folic acid.

Yogurt is naturally superior to milk in many ways. Each 8 oz serving contains 35–45% of the recommended daily calcium requirement. It is more digestible than milk. Even those who are lactose-intolerant can often eat yogurt without discomfort. There are few foods that have as many health benefits as yogurt.

Kefir is a cultured milk product that has a smaller curd size, is easier to digest, and has a more liquid consistency than yogurt. It also contains a good mixture of good bacteria and yeast; therefore, this makes a great product to add to your diet.

These studies are found in fresh yogurt and not frozen yogurt:

- The U.S. National Cancer Institute determined that malignant tumors shrink in patients who consumed a steady diet of yogurt.
- Studies at the Harvard Medical School showed that yogurt is especially effective against vaginal cancer.

Buying Yogurt

Not all yogurts are created equal. If you purchase a store-bought yogurt, then read the label carefully to make sure it contains "active cultures or live cultures." The yogurt should not contain sugars, preservatives, or thickeners. Some yogurts are produced by heat processing. This extends the shelf life but destroys the bacteria needed for health benefits. The FDA requires a "heat-treated" after cultures if this process has been used. Look for a yogurt that has a minimum of four different active cultures. It may contain up to eight active cultures; the higher the number, the better the health benefits.

In addition, note that yogurt labeled "low-fat" or "sugar free" may still contain flavorings, stabilizers, and other added chemicals. Plain low-fat yogurt is the healthiest and most digestible form.

Best option – make your own. It is easier than you would think and can be started with just a starter from a friend or bought at a good natural food store.

Adding Yogurt to Your Diet

There are many ways to incorporate yogurt into your diet. Making a healthy drink by replacing ice cream with yogurt and adding fresh or frozen fruit and honey will please any child. Yogurt also can be used in salad dressings, mashed potatoes, cole slaw, pasta salads, tuna salad, sandwich spreads, and potato salad. It can be used in place of sour cream and is great on baked potatoes. Yogurt can also be substituted for buttermilk in recipes. Don't use yogurt in cakes unless you have adjusted the leavenings.

Nondairy Yogurt

A soymilk yogurt is a healthy choice for those allergic to dairy products. The taste of these products is getting better all the time.

Making your own Sour Cream and Cream Cheese

The benefits of making your own yogurt are numerous. All you will need are a yogurt maker, milk, and yogurt starter. Follow the directions that come with your yogurt maker.

A healthy sour cream and cream cheese can be made from yogurt and a funnel or strainer. Straining 3 cups of yogurt will give you 1 cup of sour cream in 2 hours. If you continue to strain the yogurt for up to 24 hours, you will have a very healthy cream cheese.

The Donvier by Cuisipro is a Yogurt Cheese Maker that is very easy to use and can be found on many Web sites for approximately $16.

MEAT AND PROTEIN

He who eats meat eats to the Lord.

Romans 14:6 NIV

Protein/Amino Acids

PROTEIN IS ESSENTIAL to life. It:

- Is the single most important food we eat.
- Provides the structure for all living things.
- Is a necessary part of every living cell in the body.
- Makes up the greatest portion of our bodies' weight, next to water.
- Makes up muscles, ligaments, tendons, organs, glands, nails, hair, hormones, and many vital organs.
- Is needed for vitamins and minerals to be absorbed and assimilated.
- Provides energy directly to muscles.

Protein is Similar to the Alphabet

Proteins are made from amino acids. Most studies believe that there are twenty amino acids that make protein in our bodies.

Dr. Bruce Miller compares protein to the alphabet. Amino acids hook together, much like the pieces of a jigsaw puzzle, to form proteins. The twenty different amino acids combine in various ways to form our different proteins that are necessary for life. These twenty amino acids make up to 100,000 different proteins.

These numbers are difficult to visualize, so let's compare it to the alphabet. There are twenty-six different letters in the alphabet, but those letters are used to make hundreds of thousands of words in the English language. Just as those twenty-six letters are the building blocks to the alphabet, so the twenty amino acids are the building blocks for all our proteins.

These different types of proteins are made in the body as the need arises. It is necessary to have all twenty amino acids present at all times. If our daily diet does not contain all essential amino acids, then we can show signs of deficiency. These signs range from depression to indigestion to stunted growth. Without adequate protein it is like baking a cake without flour.

Protein Deficiencies

Contributors to protein deficiencies:

- Age
- Drug use
- Imbalances of other nutrients
- Impaired absorption
- Infection
- Lack of digestive enzymes
- Lack of Vitamin B
- Lack of Vitamin C
- Stress
- Trauma

Even when we get all the protein necessary in our diet, our bodies may still show signs of deficiency.

Signs of deficiency:
- Depressed immune system
- Depression
- Fatigue
- Loss of vitality
- Poor muscle tone
- Poor nail growth
- Poor wound healing
- Skin problems
- Slow or lack of growth in children
- Unusual hair loss
- Water retention

Amino Acids - Essential to virtually every function of the body

Amino acids are divided into two groups: essential and non-essential. Essential means that your body is unable to make these so they must be obtained from your diet. Non-essentials are made in your body if it is healthy.

Essential to virtually every function of the body protein works to:

- Antioxidant protection
- Build bile acids for digestion
- Detoxify chemicals
- Neurotransmitters
- Plus much, much more
- Produce hormones

Listed below are the nine essential amino acids that must be obtained in your diet and the benefits or improvements from consuming each one.

Essential Amino Acids

Histidine: Growth and repair of tissues, ulcers, digestion, gastric juices, hyperactivity, allergies, RA, anemia, production of red and white blood cells, lowers blood pressure, removes heavy metals

Isoleucine: Regulates and stabilizes blood sugar and energy levels, hemoglobin formation, increase endurance, and aid in the healing and repair of muscle tissue

Leucine: Lowers elevated blood sugar; healing of bones, muscle tissue, and skin

Valine: Hydrogen balance, muscle metabolism, tissue repair, nitrogen balance

Lysine: Proper growth and bone development; helps calcium absorption, nitrogen balance, cold sores/herpes virus; production of antibodies, hormones, enzymes; collagen formation and tissue repair; sports injuries and surgery recovery; lowers triglycerides; loss of energy, inability to concentrate, irritability, hair loss, anemia, eyes

Methionine: Toxemia, breakdown of fats, digestion, detoxification, hair, muscle weakness, osteoporosis, allergies; used to derive a brain food-choline.

Phenylanine: Depression, produces neurotransmitters, memory, learning, obesity, migraines, menstruation, arthritis, Central Nervous System

Threonine: Helps control epileptic seizures; Central Nervous System, collagen, elastin, heart, and skeletal muscle

Tryptophan: Insomnia, stabilizes moods, hyperactivity, stress, weight control, growth, hormones

Quality Protein

The best choices of protein are the ones that contain all nine essential amino acids in proper proportion. This will help build your body's health and is called "a complete protein."

Examples of complete proteins are *eggs, milk, beef, chicken, soybeans, and fish.* The problem with most of these sources is that they are high in fat and are altered by man through processing and the living conditions of the animal. As you lower the fat content in these foods, you also lower the protein content. And looking for meat without antibiotics, hormones, and sulfa drugs is difficult.

The way to get a complete protein from plant sources is to combine different foods with amino acids that complement one another. These foods lack one or more amino acids by themselves, but when combined, they make a complete protein that is healthier and easier to digest than meat. Here's a list of food combinations that will supply complete proteins:

FOODS	COMBINED WITH:
Beans	cheese, organic corn, nuts, rice, seeds, or wheat
Cornmeal	cheese, eggs, fish, lima beans, or potatoes
Legumes	any grain, nut, or seeds
Rice	beans, cheese, nuts, seeds, or wheat
Vegetables	grains, seeds, or nuts

Soy protein and quinoa are two examples of a complete protein without the need to add any other foods. Vegetables contain protein, but it would take a large amount of them to fulfill the body's protein needs.

In the Bible, Ezekiel was given a recipe to make bread that would sustain him for a long time while lying on the ground for 390 days. This bread contained all the necessary amino acids because of combining the grains and beans. After 390 days, Ezekiel was able to get up and walk away healthy.

ANIMAL FACTS--CLEAN AND UNCLEAN

The idea of clean and unclean meat was not really an issue in the days of the Old and New Testament. But today it is an object of contention. Many people believe we can eat whatever we want, but others believe we should still obey the commandments. For a full review of this topic, read week six in the *Treasures of Healthy Living Bible Study.* The study and answers may surprise you. For now, here is an overview.

A Summary of: Leviticus 11 and Deuteronomy 14

The animals established as clean and edible:

Land Animals
    a)   Divided hooves and
    b)   Chew the cud

If an animal has only one of the above, it was considered unclean.
    Examples of clean: ox, sheep, goat, deer, gazelle, antelope, etc.

Water Animals
    a)   Fins and
    b)   Scales

If an animal has only one of the above, it was considered unclean.
    Examples of clean: bass, cod, flounder, grouper, haddock, halibut, herring, salmon, mackerel, orange roughy, perch, snapper, trout, tuna, etc.

Birds and Insects
    a)   Scripture lists the birds that are edible
    b)   Winged insects with jointed legs

Examples of clean: chicken, Cornish hens, duck, quail, turkey, crickets, grasshoppers, locusts, etc.

A clean or unclean animal is defined by:

a)   **What it eats.** The *clean* animals are herbivores (plant eaters). In general, they do not eat the flesh of other animals, thereby avoiding many parasites, worms, and diseases that are in the flesh and blood of the animals. The *unclean* animals are omnivores and carnivores, eating both vegetation and animal flesh. Omnivores will, by their biological nature, eat anything.

b)   **The cleanliness of its digestive tract.** Clean animals have long digestive tracts, which are usually 10–12 times the length of their bodies. This ensures that they will completely process and eliminate toxins and poisons. Unclean animals' digestive tracts are much shorter than herbivores because the decaying flesh and by products are toxic and need to be removed from their bodies quickly.

It is important to remember that Scripture has given us guidelines to follow for the health of our bodies, and clean meats will bring the best results. But many of our meats have been altered so that they are longer beneficial to our bodies. It is very important to only choose organic, clean meats to ensure we get the most benefit to our bodies.

The clean animals that chew the cud and have divided hooves, such as the ox, sheep, goat, deer, cow, steer, buffalo, etc., because of the sacculated condition of the alimentary canal and the secondary cud and receptacle, practically have three stomachs as refining agencies and cleansing laboratories for purifying their food. This cleanses their systems of all poisonous and deleterious matter. It takes their clean vegetable food over twenty-four hours to be turned into flesh, which flesh even the pre-Mosaic law said was clean. This was not mere "ceremonious" cleansing, but it was made hygienically and physiologically clean and wholesome.

A cow's stomach contains four rumination pouches in which various kinds of bacteria help to digest grasses and grains. These bacteria compete for nutrients, crowding out harmful bacteria, viruses, and parasites. They also destroy many toxins before they reach the flesh of the cow.

In comparison, we find that the swine's anatomy, as a supplement to his bad appetite (eating any putrid thing he finds), has but one poorly constructed stomach arrangement and generally very limited excretory organs. Consequently, in about four hours after the pig has eaten his polluted swill and other putrid, offensive matter, man may eat the same second-hand off the ribs of the pig.

Cow

The healthy rumination process in a cow's digestive system gives its flesh purified nutrients and deposits of the Omega-3 fatty acids. These fatty acids (EPA) contribute towards healthy cardiovascular systems by reducing LDL cholesterol, raising HDL cholesterol, and improving the lining of blood vessels, making blood flow easier. Omega-3 fatty acids also lower blood pressure, slow the spread of breast cancers, reduce inflammation (arthritis, colitis, sinusitis, bronchitis, autoimmune disorders, etc.), and help with skin disorders and headaches. Omega-3 fatty acids are also found in fish with fins and scales, especially cold water fish such as salmon, haddock, and tuna.

Chicken

Some fowl, such as geese, ducks, chickens, and turkeys, are clean because of the gizzard that separates and cleanses all matter before it becomes flesh.

Pig

Isaiah 65:3–4 (KJV) says, "A people that provoketh me to anger continually to my face; that sacrificeth in gardens, and burneth incense upon altars of brick; Which remain among the graves, and lodge in the monuments, which eat swine's flesh, and broth of abominable things is in their vessels."

- Unclean animals are disease carriers. Pigs are known to carry up to 200 diseases and 18 different parasites and worms, including the trichinella spiralis worm, which is deadly (trichinosis). There is no known cure for this spiral worm. The trichinae worms are so small and transparent that only trained inspectors using high-powered microscopes can detect them. Just a forkful can cripple, or even kill, anyone who eats contaminated pork. Trichinosis can mimic arthritis, rheumatism, or typhoid fever.
- Pigs' digestive systems are very acidic. Pigs are gluttonous, and because of the volume of food they consume, their stomach acids become diluted, allowing all kinds of parasites, bacteria, viruses, and toxins to pass into their flesh.
- Pigs have more incidences of arthritis than any other known animal in the world. Arthritis may be a virus or a parasite transmitted from pigs to human as a result of eating their flesh and blood.
- Other worms and parasites found in the flesh of unclean swine are roundworms, gullet worms, hookworms, thorn-headed worms, trichina worms, stomach worms, nodular worms, and tapeworms.
- Even hog farmers who feed their hogs corn won't guarantee that the pigs haven't eaten rats, mice, fecal waste, or maggots.
- If swine are raised in a feed lot with other animals, such as horses, cows, etc., they will eat and drink the very refuse from these animals. This is a common occurrence on farms where the animals are not separated.
- Bacon, ham, hot dogs, pepperoni, and bologna (the "pink section" of the grocery store) are all popular choices of meat that usually come from the pig. They are loaded with sodium nitrite, which is used as a preservative. Sodium nitrate reacts with powerful acids in your stomach to form nitrosamines—one of the most potent cancer-causing agents known to man. Cancers affecting the digestive tract, such as colon, pancreatic, and stomach cancer, dominate the mortality charts. Cancer is the leading cause of death among children fourteen years old or younger, except for accidents. Sodium nitrate is so lethal that a pregnant woman can increase the risk of brain cancer in her infant by eating foods such as hotdogs.
  - Pigs are used to clean up the environment.
  - Jesus sent demons into a herd (about 2,000) of swine, sending them plunging to their deaths (Matt. 8:28–32).

Fish

And they gave him a piece of broiled fish, and of honeycomb. And he took it, and did eat before them.

Luke 24:42-43

- Scaleless fish and all shellfish are scavengers, the "garbage containers" of the waters and seas. God created these animals to clean up the waters. They are "filter feeders" that sit in one spot in shallow areas near population centers and pump water through their bodies to soak up nutrients. So along with their lunch, they often accumulate a dangerous dose of bacteria and viruses from human sewage. Shellfish are cesspools of filth, containing high levels of cholesterol, mercury, disease, worms, chemicals, and parasites.
- Shellfish can be placed in a body of water contaminated with cholera bacteria and they will purify the water. The largest cholera outbreak in the U S was in Louisiana in 1986, due to meals with shrimp, pork, vegetables, rice noodles, mussel soup, and pig blood coagulated with vinegar.
- Raw oysters, clams, and other shellfish may also harbor hepatitis.
- Deadly nerve toxins called "red tides" can strike eaters of even well-cooked shellfish. Symptoms range from paralysis to memory loss.
- The fish with scales and fins are especially rich in Omega-3 fatty acids, particularly:
  a)   DHA (Dorosahexaenoic Acid)
  b)   EPA (Eicosapentaenoic Acid)
- Scientific evidence supports the role these fats play in decreasing the risk of heart disease, inflammation, and cancer.
- In the lipids of clean fish there are alkylglycerols, which pull out any toxic mercury from its flesh. Eating this fish may allow the removal of mercury and other heavy toxic metals from our bodies as well.
- Jesus ate clean fish Himself and gave it to His disciples as well as to multitudes. (See Luke 24:42–43; John 21:9–12.)

More about Fish

And they offered him a piece of broiled fish and a honeycomb. And when he had eaten in their presence, he took what remained and gave it to them.

Luke 24:41–43 NKJ

Then, as soon as they had come to land, they saw a fire of coals there, and fish laid on it, and bread. 10 Jesus said to them, "Bring some of the fish which you have just caught."[11] Simon Peter went up and dragged the net to land, full of large fish, one hundred and fifty-three; and although there were so many, the net was not broken.

John 21:9–11 NKJ

Fishing on the Sea of Galilee and the River Jordan was a huge industry. During their exile in Egypt, the Israelites learned to prize fish from the Red Sea. For the people of the Old Testament, there were precise dietary laws for seafood: "These you may eat of all that *are* in the water: whatever in the water has fins and scales, whether in the seas or in the rivers—that you may eat. [10] But all in the seas or in the rivers that do not have fins and scales, all which move in the water or any living thing which is in the water, they *are* an abomination to you. [11] They shall be an abomination to you; you shall not eat their flesh, but you shall regard their carcasses as an abomination. [12] Whatever in the water does not have fins or scales—that *shall be* an abomination to you". Leviticus 11:9–12. NKJ

Fishy Facts:
- Thins the blood
- Protects arteries from damage
- Inhibits blood clots (anti-thrombotic)
- Strengthens the wall of the heart
- Reduces blood triglycerides
- Lowers LDL blood cholesterol
- Lowers blood pressure
- Reduces risk of heart attacks and stroke
- Eases symptoms of rheumatoid arthritis
- Reduces risk of lupus
- Relieves migraine headaches
- Fights inflammation – especially arthritis
- May help with menstrual cramps
- Helps with Psoriasis
- Prevents mood swings during post partum
- Increases mental function in Alzheimer's patients
- Helps regulate the immune system
- Inhibits cancer in animals (and possibly humans)
- Soothes bronchial asthma
- Combats early kidney disease

The key to fish's healing powers lies in the Omega-3 fatty acids, which are particularly highly concentrated in cold-water fish such as anchovies, bluefish, herring, lake trout, mackerel, sable-fish, whitefish, blue fin tuna, salmon, and sardines.

Fish oil was once something of a joke among many nutritionists. No one is laughing today about the healing powers of fish. The natural oils found in fish appear to curtail the body's overproduction of a couple of hormone-like substances called "prostaglandins" and "leukotrienes." Overactive prostaglandins and leukotrienes can cause blood clots, inflammation, and serious glitches in the immune system. Omega-3 oils halt these destructive reactions before they get out of control, something that is critical in preventing heart disease (today's number one killer).

There are three villains lurking deep inside our bodies that cause heart attacks and strokes. They are the plaque that clog arteries and dangerously restrict blood flow; the accumulation platelets (sticky pieces of blood cells) that clump together and form clots; and the sudden, unexplained spasms of blood vessels that can throw the heart out of kilter or halt the flow of blood to the brain, causing strokes. Studies on fish oil show it works wonders in reducing or eliminating all three risks. People who eat lots of fish seem to have thinner blood, which is less prone to clotting. Omega-3 oils also reduce triglycerides and dangerous LDL cholesterol and that, say the experts, may be why fish is such a powerful ally in the battle against heart disease.

Types of Fish

There are many different types of fish, some with greater potential health benefits than others. The primary health effects are linked to the level of omega-3 essential fatty acids that the fish contains. In general, fish are divided into two categories: saltwater/marine fish and freshwater fish. Recent years have seen the growth of what may be considered a third category, farm-raised fish.

Omega Content of Popular Fish Species

Highest Sources of Omega-3

FISH	GRAMS
Norway Sardines	5.1
Mackerel, Atlantic	2.6
Herring, Atlantic	1.7
Tuna, bluefish	1.6
Sablefish	1.5
Salmon, sockeye	1.3

Bluefish	1.2
Mullet	1.1
Bass, striped	0.8
Hake, silver	0.6
Pompano, Florida	0.6
Swordfish	0.2

Fishy Smell

Fish requires storage temperatures between 30– 32° F, and some store display cases reach 45° F. Many markets defrost frozen fish and sell it for fresh, letting it sit for days in their display cases. If your fish smells fishy, the fish oils are becoming rancid. Your best buy is frozen fish, because it is frozen within hours of being caught; whereas, fresh fish is often transported for days before reaching the market, unless you live in a coastal area.

To avoid the mercury content in fish, broil on a rack so that the fish is cooked above the juices that run off.

Saltwater Fish

Saltwater fish are caught in marine environments, typically oceans. All of the fish listed below are among the best to consume, as they contain good fats.

- Fatty fish include: canned sardines, mackerel, salmon, smelt, anchovies, mullet, and herring.
- Medium fat fish include: halibut, ocean perch, red snapper, sole, sea trout, and albacore tuna.
- Low-fat saltwater fish include: flounder, haddock, swordfish, cod, shellfish, and whiting.

All of the fish listed above are the best to consume, as they contain good fats.

Fresh Water Fish

Fresh water fish are caught in lakes, rivers, and streams. One concern about freshwater fish is that they may be more subject to certain types of contamination, especially high levels of mercury, depending on where they are caught. You can eliminate some of any mercury that may be present by broiling the fish on a rack so that it remains above the juices that run.

- Fatty fish includes: lake trout, mullet, smelt, and rainbow trout.

- Medium-fat fish include: carp.
- Low-fat fish include: bass, bream, pike, and Lake Perch.

Farm-Raised Fish

The omega-3 essential fatty acids found in saltwater fish come from a diet of deep-water plankton and smaller fish. Farm-raised species of fish do not appear to have as high of an omega-3 content as their wild-caught cousins. Farm-raised fish are grain fed and do not naturally produce a high omega-3 content so they are fed an omega laboratory designed diet to compensate.

- A special note about farm raised fish. If salmon are designed to live in the ocean and then travel upstream to spawn, then how are they able to live in a farm atmosphere? The answer lies in the mosquito. Chemical engineers have taken a mosquito gene and crossed it with the salmon to make the salmon able to live in a farm environment. This is called "genetic engineering."
- Never buy farm-raised fish; these are not the quality of nutrients that you are looking for in a healthy diet. Always look for fish that is caught in the wild and is fresh or freshly frozen.

"Annette's Fish Started Crawling"

Crawling fish is not Darwinism! Instead, I must tell you about a shopping trip I took to one of the favorite grocery stores here in Richmond. Usually, once in a blue moon, I can get Steve, my husband, to eat fish. Tonight was the blue moon for him. So I went and bought the fish, brought it home, seasoned it, and placed it in the refrigerator.

When time came to finish preparing dinner, I turned on the broiler and removed the prepared fish from the refrigerator. When the oven was ready, I reached for the pan of fish and noticed that something was moving! After looking more closely, I realized that my fish had given birth to creepy, crawly worms! I was shocked!

My stomach felt like I had eaten the blue moon. I quickly took my pan, searched through the trash to find the wrapper and receipt, and then took off for the grocery store. Now I must say in times like these that it is best to check out what you are wearing and if you have make-up on before running to the store, because once I arrived, I realized I was not dressed appropriately for being out of the home.

Arriving at the store, I requested to speak to the store manager and the fish department manager. The clerk said that they are one and the same—how convenient. As I showed him my dinner platter, the manager also was amazed at the continued movement. He said he didn't blame me for not wanting to eat the worms but that they are very normal. Not in my kitchen, because I am not eating fish for a very long time! His comment was that everyone eats these worms all the time in restaurants and at home; they are as natural as worms in your apples. Now tell me how many of you eat the worm in your apple—for that matter, how many of you eat the apple at all?

In case you want more information about this worm issue, in the following section I have rewritten the notes the fish manager sent me regarding this issue of Parasites in Marine Fishes!

Parasites in Marine Fishes

All living organisms, including fish, can have parasites. Parasites are a natural occurrence, not contamination. They are as common in fish as insects are in fruits and vegetables. Parasites do not present a health concern in thoroughly cooked fish.

Parasites become a concern when consumers eat raw or lightly preserved fish, such as sashimi, sushi, ceviche, and gravlax. When preparing these products, use commercially frozen fish. Alternatively, freeze the fish to an internal temperature of -4° F for at least seven days to kill any parasites that may be present. Home freezers may not be cold enough to kill the parasites.

The health risk from parasites is far less than the risk from "unseen" illness causing bacteria, which are present on almost all foods. Here are some commonly asked questions about fish parasites:

- *What are the worms that I sometimes see in fish I catch or buy?* Round worms called "nematodes" are the most common parasite found in marine fishes. Some people call these nematodes "herring worms" or "cod worms." Actually, several different species exist, and it is hard to distinguish among them. All are in the family Anisakidae and are anisakid nematodes.

    Freshwater fish like trout and fish that spend part of their life in freshwater, such as salmon, may carry Diphyllobothrium tapeworm larvae. These small, whitish, and somewhat flabby worms are common in salmon from some areas or Alaska.

- *How do fish get parasites?* The life cycle of an anisakid nematode begins when seals or sea lions eat infected fish. The larval nematodes grow to maturity, and the marine mammal excretes the nematode eggs into the sea, where they hatch. Shrimp-like animals eat the larvae, and fish eat the shrimp-like animals. The larvae then develop into the form we see in fish.

    The life cycle for a tapeworm is similar. Mammals or birds eat infected fish. The eggs hatch in freshwater. Crustaceans eat the eggs, freshwater and anadromous fish eat the crustaceans, and we eat the fish.

- *Will a parasite hurt me if I accidentally eat one?* Nematodes rarely cause health problems because they are uncommon in fish fillets and normal cooking easily destroys them. In most cases, swallowing a live nematode is harmless; the nematode passes through the intestine without causing problems.

In rare cases, swallowing a live nematode larva can cause severe gastric upset called anisakiasis. This happens when the nematode attaches to or penetrates the intestinal lining. Nematodes do not find humans to be suitable hosts and will not live longer then 7–10 days in human digestive tracts.

Swallowing live tapeworm larvae can cause a tapeworm infestation. The tape worms may live in the human intestinal tract for several years. Symptoms can include abdominal pain, weakness, weight loss, and anemia. Doctors successfully treat tapeworm infections with medicines.

- *How long should I cook fish to kill parasites?* Cooking fish to an internal temperature of 140° F will kill all fish nematodes and tapeworms. Normal cooking procedures generally exceed this temperature.

- *Are raw and lightly marinated recipes safe?* Eating raw fish, just like eating raw meat or poultry, is riskier then eating cooked products. To minimize the risk, avoid eating raw or lightly marinated seafood unless the fish is free of parasites or has been properly frozen.

- Canada's Health Protection Branch recommends using only commercially frozen fish in raw fish dishes because home freezers will not kill the parasites. The US Food and Drug Administration recommend using fish frozen commercially for seven days at -10° F.

- *Why don't processors remove parasites from fish?* Food handling practices on fishing vessels and in processing plants minimize nematode infestation. Many seafood processors inspect seafood fillets of species likely to contain parasites. Unfortunately, they cannot always see parasites embedded deep in thick fillets or in dark tissue.

- *What can consumers do if they find a worm in fish?* If a parasite is present in a fish, you have several options:

1. Remove the parasite, examine the fish for others, and cook the fish. Thorough cooking kills all parasites.

2. Notify the store where you bought the fish so that the store can carefully inspect remaining fish.

3. Depending on the return policy of the particular store, you may wish to return or exchange the unused portion.[38]

URBAN SOY MYTHS

"Boys are growing breast." "Girls are starting to menstruate at the age of six.", "Soy causes breast cancer," "I read from this doctor on his website that soy is the worst food to eat." Each week these comments are sent to my inbox along with the same question: "Why do you recommend soy as a food for us to eat?" Here I am going to explain why soy can be your best friend in nutrition and at the same time your worst enemy.

By now you are well aware of the three principles used throughout the *Treasures of Healthy Living* series; eat the foods God called food, eat foods as close to His design – before being altered, and don't let any food become your god. When it comes to soy we can answer the questions, is it a food God designed for us to eat - yes, has it been altered – very emphatically YES, and are you addicted to it – I doubt it. Since it is a food God designed then we need to understand why the controversy? The problem is complicated. Soy is a very genetically altered product and this is one main reason for the disagreement. When it is in its pure form – as God designed – we win. When it is altered – we lose. This altered state along with biased studies and misinterpreted science sends us mixed signals. Here are Dr. Stephen Chaney's (professor University North Carolina) remarks about the soy myth.

> There are a lot of "urban myths" about soy that have been repeated so often that they are widely believed to be true - even though the evidence clearly shows that they are not.
>
> It usually starts with an irresponsible blogger or web site author who likes to write sensational stories -and doesn't let the facts get in the way of a good story. They usually start out with a kernel of truth and then distort it and magnify it until it becomes unrecognizable - all in name of having a sensational story to tell. And once those stories have been repeated on many sites (without anyone bothering to do a fact check) they take on the ring of truth - and become "urban myths".
>
> For example, one of the oft-repeated urban myths is that soy protein causes breast cancer and certainly should not be used by any woman who has had breast cancer. Let's start with the "kernel of truth". Soy isoflavones bind to the estrogen receptor, and some animal experiments suggested that they might increase the risk of breast cancer. While other animal experiments came to the opposite conclusion, it was at least theoretically possible that soy protein might increase the risk of breast cancer and might be contraindicated for women with estrogen sensitive breast cancer. Of course, it is a far cry from saying that this is a theoretical possibility to the dire warnings that appeared on some web sites.
>
> Of course, whenever a hypothesis like this surfaces, the best way to resolve the question is through clinical studies. Three major clinical studies have been published in the last few years showing that soy protein consumption reduces - not increases - the risk of breast cancer.

The most compelling of these was a recent study reported in the Journal of the American Medical Association (302: 2437-2443, 2009). That study looked at women who had already had breast cancer and showed that soy protein consumption significantly decreased the likelihood of breast cancer recurrence - even in those women with estrogen sensitive breast cancer. That study also showed that soy protein did not interfere with the estrogen blocking drug tamoxifen. In fact, it enhanced tamoxifen activity.

Unfortunately, none of the originators of the soy-breast cancer warning have seen fit to alter their web sites based on the actual clinical data, so this urban myth persists.

Another urban myth is that soy protein consumption will affect male fertility. The "kernel of truth" here is that soy isoflavones also resemble testosterone. My first take on this has always been that if soy affects male fertility, someone obviously forgot to tell the Chinese. More to the point, several recent clinical studies have shown that soy protein consumption does not affect testosterone levels, sperm count or any other measure of male fertility.

And, of course, there is always the myth that soy protein consumption affects serum thyroid levels. The "kernel of truth" here is that when taken simultaneously with thyroid medication, soy protein - and many other foods - decreases absorption of the medication. However, numerous clinical studies have shown that soy protein has no effect on endogenous serum thyroid hormone levels and does not interfere with thyroid medication if taken 30-60 minutes later.

By now, many of you are probably wondering when I will get around to talking about soy protein isolate. So let me get off my soapbox and address the topic of the day. I received an "urgent" email from someone last week saying that they had read that soy protein isolate was treated with strong acid, strong alkali, heated to very high temperatures and was loaded with MSG. While some of those statements can be true for hydrolyzed soy protein, none of them are true for soy protein isolate.

The first step in preparation of soy protein isolate is to remove impurities with either an alcohol or water washing process. The water washing process is preferable because it preserves the important soy isoflavones. Next the protein is precipitated out of solution by adding just enough dilute acid to bring the pH to 4-5. To put that in perspective, that is 100-fold less acidic than a soft drink, 10-fold less acidic than an orange and slightly less acidic than a strawberry. Finally, enough dilute alkali is added to bring the pH back to neutrality (pH7). None of this requires high temperatures, and no MSG is released in the process.

Where is the "kernel of truth" here? I'm not sure, but I suspect that the original web site authors or bloggers were confusing soy protein isolate with hydrolyzed soy protein.

The term hydrolyzed soy protein or soy protein hydro lysate simply means that the purified soy protein has been hydrolyzed to the individual amino acids. This can involve treating the soy protein with strong acid at high temperature, but it can also involve treating the soy protein with proteases (enzymes that hydrolyze proteins) at low temperatures. In either case, this step will be followed by adding just enough alkali to bring the amino acids back to neutral pH. If you are consuming a food or supplement containing hydrolyzed soy protein you might wish to see if you can find out which process they use.

The hydrolysis process will release MSG (the sodium salt of the amino acid glutamic acid) along with the sodium salt of all the other amino acids. Because this same process occurs in our intestines when we digest any protein, it is not clear that the MSG contained in a protein hydro lysate is as harmful as extra MSG added as a flavor enhancer to foods. That remains a theoretical possibility. We'll just need to wait for clinical studies to see if it is a real concern.

Hopefully, these tips from Professor Chaney will help you separate soy myths from soy facts. The other problem is not only the soy opponents but the soy manufacturers who make claims that go beyond the clinical studies. So as is true of everything you consume: follow the three principles and make principle two – eat the foods as close to the way God designed as possible – your main mantra for eating.

Soy Fighting Estrogen's Effects

By acting as weak estrogens, according to the American Institute for Cancer Research, isoflavones possibly substitute for estrogens at certain cellular sites, providing beneficial effects. They may act as anti-estrogens, preventing the hormone from wielding its cancer-promoting effects. This theory may clarify why high-soy diets have been linked specifically to lower risks of hormone-related cancers, says the AICR. It would also help to explain why soy seems to demonstrate health benefits at a number of sites in the body.

Estrogen receptor sites can be likened to docks at a port; if a ship is already docked, another cannot take its place. Isoflavones work in very much the same way; if a site is occupied by a phytoestrogen, then estrogen simply won't dock on that particular cell. If enough soy isoflavones are circulating in the body, the majority of these sites (located in the breast, prostate, uterus, and colon areas) will remain occupied by beneficial isoflavones. "The anti-estrogenic potential of isoflavones includes their ability to compete with or bind estrogen receptors, thereby preventing the action of the body's own estrogens," says Holt. "Genistein, which has only 1/1000 the hormonal activity of estrogen attaches to the estrogen receptors, blocking the more potent female hormone from attaching itself to these vulnerable sites."

In addition to its anticancer properties, soy isoflavones function as antioxidants, which seek and destroy damaging molecules that have the ability to impair immunity. Like other antioxidants, soy can reduce long-term risk of cancer and other chronic diseases by preventing free radical damage.

Clinical studies documenting the benefits of soy are overwhelmingly conclusive; it works health wonders. Those wonders are turning more and more people to soy.

THE SOY TRUTH

by Dr. Richard Brouse

Common Concerns about Soy:

1. *Do soybeans cause cancer?* It is true that "overcooked" soy contains "carcinogenic" compounds. When soy is extruded through high temperature, high-pressure steam nozzles to form what is called "textured vegetable protein –TVP for short," this form of processing renders the soy "meat substitute" carcinogenic or cancer causing. TVP is what is used in soy dogs and soy burgers, and should be avoided.

2. *What about roasted soybeans?* Whole soybeans are high in plant fat. If soybeans are roasted to eat as soy nuts, the heat alters the fat and makes it a trans-fatty acid, which causes both cancer and heart disease. As roasted soy nuts sit on the shelf or in the cupboard in storage, the oils are becoming more and more rancid and carcinogenic. Avoid roasted soybeans.

3. *But I've heard that soy protein is hard on the kidneys!* Animal protein is much harder to digest than vegetable protein. Since many people have digestive difficulties, protein not thoroughly digested is very challenging to the kidneys. Powdered protein is in a predigested state, and the best protein source to choose! Protein is not the enemy—it is essential for life. It is true; however, that excessive protein is hard on the kidneys. So if a person consumes more than two grams of protein per pound of body weight daily and does not consume adequate carbohydrates with it, this could cause kidney damage.

4. *I have breast cancer, and I've been told I cannot have soy!* It is true that soy is a "phyto-estrogen" food, which means it contains substances that have hormone-like components. However, their estrogen strength is 1/1000th that of the body's own stronger estrogens. Therefore, you want to load your digestive system with quality controlled raw soy powder, because these weaker estrogens will block the estrogen receptor sites from receiving your body's own stronger estrogens and therefore be very protective against estrogen fed cancer.

Essential Seven Checklists for a Quality Soy Product:

1. *Were the soybeans ORGANICALLY GROWN?* Studies have shown decreased levels of food nutrients and increased levels of nitrates in chemically fertilized crops, when compared with their organic counterparts. There is a connection between the ingestion of nitrates and cancer! Therefore, it is important to know that pesticides, fungicides, and herbicides have not been used during the growing process. In particular, with soybeans, since they are such a hardy plant, a powerful and deadly weed spray called Round-Up is usually used. For your safety, you must know that your soy products are organically grown.

2. *Were the soybeans genetically engineered?* Genetically engineered soybeans are much cheaper to purchase, and most companies producing soy products look for ways to save money.

3. *Does your soybean powder contain all of the nine essential amino acids?* One of the most valuable features of the soybean is that it is a complete protein and provides all nine of the essential amino acids. The body requires these daily to produce hormones, digestive juices, antibodies, and enzymes. However, not all soybeans are created equal. Quality and amino acid content will vary based on soil conditions and variable growing and harvest conditions. If one essential amino acid is missing, the immune system can be depressed 30%, and many important body functions are delayed or stopped. Therefore, it is essential that each batch of soybeans be checked for amino acid content if we want to depend on the soy isolate to provide a guaranteed supply of the nine essential amino acids.

4. *Were the crushed soy flakes washed in alcohol or water?* Alcohol washing destroys isoflavones content up to 88%! It is the isoflavones that reduce the risk of breast, prostate, lung, and bowel cancer. Also, it is the isoflavones that are so beneficial in hormone balancing and increasing bone mass.

5. *Was the "anti-thyroid," "anti-growth" substance in the raw soy removed?* Orientals, who

have consumed large amounts of soy for years, have known that *raw* soy contains an "anti-growth," "anti-tyrosine" substance. Tyrosine deficiency will cause low blood pressure, low body temperature, and restless leg syndrome. Therefore, Orientals always lightly cook their soy foods to deactivate the "anti-tyrosine/anti-growth" substance. Shaklee has designed an extracting process that removes this substance yet keeps the soy in a raw form in order to maintain the highest level of amino and isoflavones, which are very sensitive to heat.

6. *Is your soybean food raw or heated?* Amino acids are very sensitive to heat. In some studies, cooking protein has been shown to destroy up to 50% of some essential amino acids. If an individual consistently consumes a diet that is lacking in all of the essential amino acids, inadequate brain development and hormones or other body tissue development can be the result.

7. *Has calcium been added to your soy powder?* Some negative reports about soy say that soy powders are very acidic and cause bone loss because it causes calcium to be drawn from the bones. The raw soy bean is a neutral food—neither acidic nor alkaline. However, the removal of the soybean oil (which is essential so that the soy powder will not go rancid very quickly) makes the powder very acidic. Therefore, adequate calcium (which is very alkaline) must be added to cause the powder to be neutral again, or it can cause the above-stated problem. Many protein powder manufacturers do not add any or enough calcium.

SWEET DESIGN

How Sweet Is It?

The average American consumes an astounding two to three pounds of sugar each week. That's about 140 pounds a year and does not take into account the amount of high fructose corn syrup consumed which would increase this total to as much as 220 pounds per year in some people. This is not surprising, considering that high levels of sugar being processed into such foods as bread, breakfast cereal, mayonnaise, peanut butter, spaghetti sauce, and microwave meals.

Prior to the turn of this century, sugar consumption was only five pounds per person per year. Cardiovascular disease was virtually unknown in the early 1900s. In the last twenty years, we have increased sugar consumption to those 220 pounds of sugar per person per year, which averages about eighteen pounds a month or 62 teaspoons a day!

Effects of Sugar on Your Health

Sugar:

- Can cause eczema in children.
- Can cause toxemia during pregnancy.
- Causes a rise in triglycerides.
- Causes drowsiness and decreased activity.
- Causes food allergies.
- Causes free radical damage in the bloodstream.
- Causes headaches, including migraines.
- Causes hormonal imbalance.
- Causes hypertension.

- Causes hypoglycemia.
- Causes kidney damage.
- Contributes to diabetes.
- Contributes to hyperactivity, anxiety, depression, concentration difficulties, and crankiness in children.
- Contributes to osteoporosis.
- Contributes to weight gain and obesity.
- Increases blood platelet adhesiveness, which causes blood clots and strokes.
- Increases the amount of fat in the liver.
- Increases the body's fluid retention.
- Increases the risk of Coronary Heart disease.
- Increases the risk of Crohn's Disease and ulcerative colitis.
- Increases total cholesterol.
- Interferes with absorption of calcium and magnesium.
- Leads to chromium deficiency.
- Leads to Periodontal disease.
- Produces an acidic stomach.
- Promotes tooth decay.
- Raises adrenaline levels in children.
- Speeds the aging process, causing wrinkles.
- Suppresses the immune system for 4 hours.
- Upsets the body's mineral balance.
- Weakens defenses against bacterial infections.

Sweeteners to Avoid

When we understand that we have a portion of our tongues made primarily to enjoy sweets, we realize that all sweets are not bad for us. It is important to remember to enjoy all food in the way it was created and before it is altered by man. The list here is about sweeteners that have been altered by man. As you read this list and the effects of using these substitutes, it makes perfect sense to only eat the foods created by an Almighty God.

NutraSweet/Aspartame

Know the Facts: aspartame (NutraSweet/Equal) is a synthetic chemical used in place of sugar. It consists of Aspartic Acid, Phenylalanine, and methanol (methyl alcohol). This is why it had to be approved by the FDA; it is a drug!

Do not use this if you are pregnant, lactating, or have phenylketonura. For more information, see the in-depth information on aspartame in this manual.

Saccharin (Sweet N Low, Sugar Twin)

This is made from a chemical similar to acesulfame-K, which is 350 times sweeter than sugar. It has been on the market for over sixty years, but its safety still has not been established. Animal studies have shown an increased risk of bladder cancer, which prompted an attempt to ban the sweetener. The move was thwarted by Congress to appease consumers. They decided to add a warning label instead. It is still on a government list of "likely" carcinogens.

Do not use saccharin if pregnant or lactating, and do not give it to children.

Acesulfame–K (Sunnett)

This is a nonnutritive sweetener that is 200 times sweeter than regular table sugar. It is not metabolized, so it has no calories. Acesulfame-K is used in chewing gum, instant coffee, tea, dry beverage mixes, gelatins, and nondairy creamers. The CSPI (Center for Science in the Public Interest) objects to this chemical since it caused an increase growth of tumors in rats. The FDA concluded that the tumors had occurred spontaneously.

Sucralose (Splenda)

Approved in 1998, sucralose is a non-calorie sweetener made from real sugar. Scientists alter the structure of the sugar molecule, making it much sweeter than sugar. Since it has been on the market for over eight years, there have been many studies completed to show that this altering does in fact cause health risks. Read more about this on the section entitled "Splenda: What You Need to Know."

Alitame (Aclame)

This is a candidate for approval as an artificial sweetener. It has 2,000 times the sweetness of sugar and no calories. It can potentially be used in all products. It is derived from the amino acid alanine and related to aspartame.

Cyclamate

This was an artificial sweetener made from sodium and calcium. It was thirty times sweeter than sugar. It was removed from the market in 1969 since it was found to cause various cancers. There has been a concerted effort to bring cyclamates back to the market, but as of 2010, it has not been approved. According to www.clyclamate.org, a China based company supplying the world wide product states that Abbott Laboratories is still petitioning the FDA to allow it on the U.S. market.

Neotame

On July 9, 2002, the FDA approved the general use of this chemical as a flavor enhancer and sweetener. It is made by the same company as aspartame in Illinois. Neotame, like aspartame, contains aspartic acid, phenylalanine, and a methyl ester. Neuroscientists have found that aspartic acid and glutamic acid load on the same receptors in the brain, cause identical brain lesions and neuroendocrine disorders, and act in an addictive fashion. People who are sensitive to MSG and/or aspartame will have similar effects when ingesting neotame.

No artificial sweetener should play a major role in a healthful diet. *Stevia is the only sugar substitute that does not have the possibility of negatively affecting your health.* Read Labels. Wiser choices will be the natural sweeteners God gave us to enjoy sparingly.

NutraSweet/Aspartame: An In-Depth Analysis

Know the Facts:

- Thirty years ago, a chemist searching for a medicine to relieve ulcers accidentally discovered the chemical combination we now know as aspartame. Sold under names like NutraSweet and Equal, what was intended as a drug has become a food additive that is used in larger quantities and by more people, from tiny babies to the elderly, than any one person would ever use a prescription medicine.

- Once listed in the Pentagon's inventory of prospective biochemical-warfare weapons, aspartame is a volatile combination of chemicals—Aspartic Acid, Phenylanine, and methanol—the most lethal being methanol or wood alcohol. The Random House Dictionary defines methanol, also known as methyl alcohol, as "a colorless, poisonous liquid used chiefly as a solvent, fuel, etc."

- Methanol is what is called a cumulative poison. In other words, it is a toxic substance that your body never eliminates. Instead, it builds up over time, wreaking havoc with your nervous system and causing all kinds of potential other problems. It could even lead to death.

  Methanol can be a deadly metabolic poison, which converts to formaldehyde and then to formic acid (deadly). One of the reasons methanol is so toxic is because the body lacks the necessary enzymes to detoxify it.

  Furthermore, the body is unable to assimilate the large quantity of Phenylalanine and Aspartic Acid. These amino acids can become neurotoxin (poisonous to nerves), deteriorating and killing brain cells!

- Every time you ingest something that is artificially sweetened, whether it's a toothpaste, soft drink, or dessert, you are consuming poisonous wood alcohol. A full 10% of each and every NutraSweet molecule is made up of Methanol, more than

1,000 times greater than most foods under FDA control.
- When aspartame is consumed, especially in beverages, the body is suddenly deluged with large amounts of phenylalanine and aspartic acid, which can cross into the brain unopposed and cause significant disturbances of the brain neurotransmitter and endocrine functions.
- Only fifty studies on humans and 100 studies on animals were done to test the safeness of aspartame.
- Sold in over 5,000 products internationally, including soft drinks, breath mints, gum, Jell-O, lemonade, milk drinks, children's vitamins, lollipops, yogurt, pudding, instant breakfast, and anything that says Low Fat or Sugar-Free (unless it is using Splenda—read about that).
- The quickest way to get aspartame to the brain is through chewing gum.
- The recommended limit of consumption is 7.8 mg/day. A large serving of aspartame would be equal to 4 sodas per day. Remember a serving is 8 ounces and most food stores/ restaurants/ gas stations serve larger than 8 ounce servings. This makes it easy to ingest more then the safe limit.
- Scientists believe aspartame will "trigger" or "worsen" the symptoms of Multiple Sclerosis, Fibromyalgia, Alzheimer's, Parkinson's, Systemic Lupus, and Thyroid Disorders.
- The effects of aspartame are documented by the FDA's own data. In 1995 the agency was forced, under the Freedom of Information Act, to release a list of ninety-two aspartame symptoms reported by thousands of victims. It appears this is only the tip of the iceberg. H. J. Roberts, M.D., published the medical text "Aspartame Disease: An Ignored Epidemic." This contains 1,000 pages of symptoms and diseases triggered by this neurotoxin and includes the sordid history of its approval.

Aspartame Side Effects
- Abnormal Brain Function
- Anxiety Attacks
- Arrhythmias
- Blindness
- Death
- Dizziness
- Fatigue
- Gastrointestinal disorders
- Headaches
- Heart Attack Symptoms
- Hyperactivity

- Insomnia
- Insomnia
- Loss of Taste
- Migraines
- Mood Swings
- Muscle Spasms
- Numbness
- Personality Changes
- PMS
- Possible Birth Defects
- Ringing in the Ears
- Seizures (80% increase, especially in children)
- Severe Depression
- Slurred Speech
- Tachycardia
- Weight Gain

Excitotoxins, The Taste that Kills, by Russell L. Blaylock, M.D., is a well-written and thoroughly researched book on the topic of aspartame. This reading explains how the brain is affected by chemicals in our food such as aspartame and MSG. I highly recommend reading this book to get a better understanding.

NOT SO SPLENDID SPLENDA

Splenda is another name for sucralose, a synthetic compound stumbled upon in 1976 by scientists in Britain who were seeking a new pesticide formulation. Splenda is a chlorocarbon. Chlorocarbons long have been known for causing organ, genetic, and reproductive damage. For example, chlorocarbons can cause up to 40% shrinkage of the thymus, a gland that is the very foundation of our immune system; the swelling of the liver and kidneys; and calcification of the kidneys.

Research in animals has shown that sucralose can cause many problems, such as:

- Shrunken thymus glands
- Enlarged liver and kidneys
- Atrophy of lymph follicles in the spleen and thymus
- Reduced growth rate
- Decreased red blood cell count
- Hyperplasia of the pelvis

- Extension of the pregnancy period
- Aborted pregnancy
- Decreased fetal body weights and placental weights
- Diarrhea

As you seek to improve your health by using the guidelines for choosing foods designed by God—not altered and not addicting—it is easy to see that Splenda is an altered product that can lead you to an addiction of food containing it.

While some industry experts claim the molecule is similar to table salt or sugar, other independent researcher's say that it has more in common with pesticides. That's because the bonds holding the carbon and chlorine atoms together are more characteristic of a chlorocarbon than a salt—and most pesticides are chlorocarbons.

The premise offered next is that just because something contains chlorine, that doesn't guarantee it's toxic. And that is also true; but you and your family may prefer not to serve as test subjects for the latest post-market artificial sweetener experiment—however "unique."

So, is Splenda safe?

The truth is we just don't know yet. There are no long-term studies of the side effects of Splenda in humans. The manufacturer's own short-term studies showed that sucralose caused shrunken thymus glands and enlarged livers and kidneys in rodents. But in this case, the FDA decided that because these studies weren't based on humans, they were not conclusive. Of course, there are countless examples of foods and drugs that have proven dangerous to humans that were first found to be dangerous to laboratory rats, and then again, countless others that have not. So the reality is that we are the test subjects for Splenda.

Splenda Side Effects

Observational evidence shows that there are side effects of Splenda, including skin rashes/flushing, panic-like agitation, dizziness and numbness, diarrhea, muscle aches, headaches, intestinal cramping, bladder issues, and stomach pain. These show up at one end of the spectrum—in the people who have an allergy or sensitivity to the sucralose molecule. It appears that no one is sure to what degree consuming Splenda affects the rest of us.

If this sounds familiar, it should, because we went down the same path with aspartame, the main ingredient in Equal and NutraSweet. Almost all of the independent research into aspartame found dangerous side effects in rodents. The FDA chose not to take these findings into account when it approved aspartame for public use. Over the course of fifteen years, those same side effects increasingly appeared in humans. Not in everyone, of course, but in those who were vulnerable to the chemical structure of aspartame.

As food additives, artificial sweeteners are not subject to the same gauntlet of FDA safety trials as pharmaceuticals. Most of the testing is funded by the food industry, which has a vested interest in the outcome. This can lead to misleading claims on both sides.

But one thing is certain: some of the chemicals that comprise artificial sweeteners are known hazards. The degree to which you experience side effects just depends on your individual biochemistry. Manufacturers are banking on the fact that our bodies won't absorb very much of these compounds at any one time. And many of us don't. But what happens when we are ingesting artificial sweeteners like Splenda dozens of times a week through many different "low-sugar" or "sugar-free" products?

People have been using artificial sweeteners for decades. Some react poorly, some don't. The problem is that you never know until you're already sick. Scientists are calling Splenda a mild mutagen, based on how much is absorbed. Right now, it's anyone's guess what portion of the population is being exposed to the dangers of Splenda or already suffering from Splenda's side effects. Until an independent, unbiased research group conducts long-term studies on humans (six months is hardly long-term!), how can we be certain?

With all the new Splenda products on our shelves, it looks as if we are now in the process of another grand public experiment—without our permission. And we may not know the health implications for decades. As with all things, time will unveil truth.

RECOGNIZING NATURAL SWEETENERS

Agave Nectar

Agave is a sweet syrup, like honey, but a little thinner in consistency. Because it has a low glycemic index and will not elevate blood sugar, it is a great honey replacement for diabetics and low-glycemic dieters.

Agave nectar is made from the juice of Agave Tequilana, the same variety of agave that is processed into the alcoholic drink tequila. The agave plant is considered the "Mexican Tree of Life and Abundance" and was a favorite food of the Aztecs. Agave nectar is a wonderful sweetener for beverages such as ice tea or lemonade, as it dissolves easily. Drizzle it over yogurt or cereal. Use it to sweeten salad dressings and BBQ sauce. For baking, you can substitute agave in recipes just as you would substitute honey. Use three-fourths agave for the recommended amount of sugar and reduce the amount of liquid.

Be cautious when purchasing this sweetener; it is rumored that some products include very little agave and have high fructose corn syrup as a filler. Verify the source of the company you are purchasing from before making this purchase. Xagave is one of the better brands on the market.

Apple Syrup

Apple syrup is made by cooking down apple cider until it reaches a consistency like maple syrup. It can be used like maple syrup. It has a strong apple flavor.

Barley Malt Syrup

This is a liquid sweetener that is reminiscent of molasses. It can be substituted for molasses in baking. Barley malt syrup metabolizes slowly in the body but does have calories and carbohydrates. Diabetics and low-carbohydrate dieters should use it with caution. Otherwise, it is fine for anyone who wants a whole-food natural sweetener. Barley malt syrup is considered to be one of the healthiest sweeteners in the natural food industry, since it is produced from a whole food source and is made of the simple sugars.

Birch Syrup

Birch syrup is similar to maple syrup in that it is tapped from a tree and boiled down to concentrate the sugar. Currently it is harvested only in very small quantities from paper birch trees in Alaska's boreal forests.

It takes an average of 100 gallons of sap to make 1 gallon of birch syrup. (Maple syrup requires 40 gallons of sap to make 1 gallon of syrup.) The sap contains only 1–1.5% sugar and looks and tastes much like water right out of the tree.

Birch syrup is high in vitamins and minerals, including vitamin C, potassium, manganese, thiamin, and calcium. It has "a rich, spicy-sweet flavor" and is recommended for use in marinades, barbecue sauces, dressings, baked beans, coffee, baked squash, baked goods, breads, milkshakes, natural sodas, and ice cream.

Brown Rice Syrup

Brown rice syrup is a liquid sweetener with the consistency of honey. It can be substituted for honey in baking. It has a unique caramel-like flavor that can be used to enhance a recipe, but it will disappear if used sparingly in a recipe.

Brown rice syrup metabolizes slowly but does have calories and carbohydrates. Diabetics and low-carbohydrate dieters should use it with caution. Otherwise, it is fine for anyone who wants a whole-food natural sweetener.

Brown rice syrup is made by combining barley malt and brown rice and cooking the mixture until all the starch is converted to sugar. It is only 20% as sweet as sugar.

This syrup is considered to be one of the healthiest sweeteners in the natural food industry, since it is produced from a whole food source and is made of the simple sugars.

Brown rice syrup is excellent for a bit of sweetness on toast, whole grains, sweet potatoes or squash, or in tea. It blends well to sweeten salad dressings, soups, and sauces.

Corn Syrup

This is a sweetener you will find listed on many labels. Corn syrup is a highly processed sweetener that contributes to a high sweet taste in processed foods which leads to overeating. The corn, wheat and soy plants in America are genetically engineered to withstand a large amount of pesticides on the plant during growing season. For this reason alone it is best to only consume organic corn, wheat, and soy products. That would include corn syrup and high fructose corn syrup.

Dates and Date Sugar

Dates are simply the fruit of various varieties of palm trees. Date sugar is made by simply dehydrating dates and grinding them up into a rather coarse, granulated-type sugar. It contains fiber and nutrients, just as fresh dates do. Although it will not dissolve very well in your cup of coffee, it works very well, substituted cup for cup, in any baked-goods recipe that calls for brown sugar.

Though fresh dates score low on the glycemic index, dried fruits always score higher. And dehydration would make the score higher still, as the sugar becomes more and more concentrated. So date sugar is not recommended for diabetics or those on a low-glycemic diet. But it's great for anyone else who wants a very unrefined close-to-nature sweetener.

Evaporated Cane Juice, Sucanat, Savannah Gold, Honey Crystals

"Evaporated organic cane juice" is just that—the juice of the same sugar cane used to make refined white sugar, but in its whole, almost natural state. Only the water is removed. As a whole food, it still retains many vitamins and minerals. It also retains its natural balance of sucrose, glucose, and fructose instead of being straight sucrose.

Sucanat Natural is typically the darker-colored sucanat, containing molasses. Sucanat with Honey or Savannah Gold is a lighter-colored sucanat, containing honey. Both are used to replace sugar cup for cup.

Fruit Spreads

Fruit spreads are like jam or preserves, but they are sweetened with concentrated fruit juice syrup instead of sugar. Usually these syrups are made from grape, apple, pear, or pineapple juice, or some combination of these. These are all natural, unrefined fructose. They are delicious and taste even better than the sugar-sweetened variety because the sweetener is more harmonious in character with the natural fruit.

Unfortunately, the fruit spreads that contain organic fruit are sweetened with sugar, and the natural fruit spreads are sweetened with fruit. I haven't yet found a fruit spread that is fruit-sweetened and made with organic fruit.

Be sure to read labels carefully, as some brands sell both sugar-sweetened and fruit-sweetened spreads and you can't tell which is which from the front label.

Fruitsource

This is a relatively new sweetener that comes in a granular and syrup form. It is made from grape juice and whole brown rice and considered to be a complex carbohydrate. It can be used like honey or any type of sugar.

Honey

Honey is "the nectar and floral exudations of plants gathered and stored in the comb of honeybees." Honey is a thick, sticky syrup that is 40% sweeter than sugar. It comes in a wide range of colors and flavors. Darker honeys have stronger flavors and lighter honeys more mild flavors. Honey has many health benefits, particularly when eaten raw.

Honey is in perfect edible form in its natural state, requiring no processing. It was one of our first sweeteners and highly prized around the world for centuries. It was our primary sweetener until the industrialization of sugar cane in the mid-1800s. In its filtered form, it should be considered the same as refined sugar. Purchase raw, unpasteurized honey. Sage and Tupelo honey breakdown more slowly in the blood stream and are a healthier choice for diabetics.

Maple Syrup

Maple syrup is a very sweet, liquid sweetener made by harvesting the sap from maple trees and boiling it down to syrup. As continued boiling removes even more water, it turns into that nice, creamy maple sugar candy, and eventually into granules. It has its own unique flavor that is well-known and well-loved.

Maple syrup and maple sugar have a very high glycemic index and will make your blood sugar jump. If you are diabetic or if you are on a low-glycemic diet, it is best to avoid maple syrup. It's fine for anyone else who wants a very low-processed natural sweetener.

Purchase maple syrup that is pure and free from formaldehyde. There are two varieties—A and B. The A is usually a milder taste and better for pancakes.

Black Strap Molasses

Blackstrap molasses is a byproduct of refining sugar. It contains about 50% sugar, as well as minerals and vitamins separated during the refining. It is rich in calcium, potassium, iron, B vitamins, and minerals, and lacks none of the essential nutrients that other forms of sugar are often deficient in. It is one of the best natural sweeteners, and it is even used in infant formulas.

Raw Sugar or Turbinado

This is just slightly less refined than table sugar and has little nutritional value.

Stevia

Stevia is one of the few natural sweeteners that has the same characteristics as an artificial sweetener—it has no calories and will not elevate blood sugar, yet it is super-sweet. It is one of the best natural sweeteners available. Many health benefits have been attributed to stevia, both in traditional use and recent scientific studies.

Stevia rebaudiana is a naturally sweet plant native to South America. It is a perennial herb of the composite family, related to lettuce, marigold, and chicory. The sweetness and taste of stevia products differ, according to the conditions under which the plant is grown and how it is processed.

The most popular and useful forms of stevia are the powdered extract or a clear liquid. These are *very, very, very* sweet, so a little goes a long way. Stevia can be used to sweeten a variety of foods, however, you cannot substitute it cup for cup or even teaspoon for teaspoon for sugar. Cooking with it takes some familiarity and practice. Typically, one teaspoon of Stevia is equal to 1 cup of sugar.

Stevia is heat stable to 392 degrees F, which makes it ideal as a sweetener to be added to any hot beverage. The liquid or extract powders will easily dissolve in cold drinks. Small bottles of stevia liquid and packets of powder are easy to carry with you as an alternative to the sugar and artificial sweeteners in restaurants.

The difficulty in using stevia as a primary sweetener is that it cannot be easily substituted for white sugar. Because so little stevia is used, it does not have the "bulk" of white sugar, which is often as crucial to a recipe as the sweetness. And stevia does not have the same physical properties as sugar, so it cannot be used, for example, to make candy. But it's fine to use when all you need is sweetness, such as to sweeten whipped cream or a salad dressing.

Truvia

Truvia is the newest sweetener in town, and has three ingredients on the label: Erythritol, rebina and natural flavors. Erythritol is made from GMO corn, rebina is derived from the stevia plant and natural flavors – well who knows what this is. So bottom line – avoid the unknown.

Vegetable Glycerin

Vegetable glycerin is derived from palm (coconut) oil. It is colorless, odorless, does not make blood sugar rise, and is about half again sweeter than sugar. It is a liquid used in many cosmetic preparations and in commercial food preparation, but it is not yet widely sold as a sweetener. Your natural food store may carry it, or you can order it online.

Manitol, Sorbitol, and Xylitol

These sweeteners are all naturally-occurring sugar alcohols. Manitol is the least common sugar alcohol used in the food industry. Diabetics use sorbitol because it is absorbed slowly and does not elevate blood sugar levels rapidly. Xylitol looks and tastes a lot like white sugar and can replace white sugar in most recipes cup for cup. It has the same sweetness and bulk as cane sugar, with one-third fewer calories. Xylitol is metabolized independently from insulin and is slowly absorbed, making it a low-glycemic sweetener, safe for diabetics. The white crystalline powder is made from plants such as birch and other hard wood trees and fibrous vegetation such as corn cobs.

As mentioned above, Xylitol is a naturally-occurring sugar alcohol; it is not a sugar. The sweetener is found in many foods, including fruits, berries, mushrooms, and lettuce. It is not a strange or artificial substance to our bodies, but it is a normal part of everyday metabolism.

Xylitol has many health benefits, including preventing cavities and many types of infections. It has been used since the 1960s in foods such as chewing gum, gum drops, and hard candy and in pharmaceuticals and oral health products such as throat lozenges, cough syrups, children's chewable multivitamins, toothpastes, and mouthwashes. However, it was not marketed as a sweetener because the price was twenty times that of sugar. Lower prices now have made it possible to make xylitol available to the home cook.

The safety of Xylitol has been proven in long-term clinical studies. It is approved as a sweetener in more than thirty-five countries. The World Health Organization and the FDA have given Xylitol their safest ratings for food additives. Babies and small children can use it without restriction. But families with pets – foods made with Xylitol should not be given to pets.

Sweet conclusion: When whole foods containing any of these sugars are consumed, the foods also provide vitamins, minerals, and proteins, stabilizing the blood sugar and aiding in digestion. When fruit is eaten, the fructose is diluted by large portions of water and fiber contained in the fruit. Refined sugars are void of the nutrients as well as the fiber and can create many health problems.

Honey

And he put forth the end of the rod, and dipped it in the honeycomb. And he carried his hand to his mouth and his eyes were enlightened.

1 Samuel 14:27 NKJ

My son, eat honey, for it is good; and the honeycomb which is sweet to your taste.

Proverbs 24:13 NKJ

For many reasons—mostly because it tastes so good—honey was one of the most popular foods among the people of the Bible. It became a symbol for abundance and God's blessings, thus, "a land flowing with milk and honey" Exodus 3:8.

What is Honey?

Unlike table sugar, which is 99.5 percent sucrose, raw honey is a natural sweetener made up of at least 165 identifiable components. It contains amino acids, enzymes, vitamins, minerals, and at least twenty-five different kinds of sugar. A list of these nutrients can be found on the Designed Healthy Living Web site (http://designedhealthyliving.com).

The exact composition of honey varies, depending upon the nectars from which it is made. For example, bees collecting nectar from buckwheat blossoms produce a dark, strong-flavored honey that is richer in minerals than the mode, white honey collected from clover blossoms.

The sugars in honey are also varied. Unlike table sugar, which, as mentioned above, is almost pure sucrose, honey contains several simple sugars. All of the sugars are the result of enzymes that bees add to the nectar they collect. The enzymes break down the raw sugars in nectar and rearrange their components into a wide variety of new sugars.

As a foraging bee returns to the hive, it passes on its drop of nectar to other bees, which "ripen" the honey further. Eventually, a worker bee spreads the drop of nectar as a thin film on the floor of an empty honeycomb cell to evaporate. When the water content reaches 20% or less, other bees continue filling the cell with nectar. When it is full, they seal it with an airtight wax cap.

Honey has a complex nature; at least eleven disaccharides are present in honey, in addition to the monosaccharide. These disaccharides include maltose, isomaltose, nigerose, turanose, and maltulose. In fact, honey is such a complex substance that, when eaten in moderate amounts, it contributes to the metabolic balance of our bodies rather than detracting from it.

Health Benefits of Honey:

- Calms frayed nerves
- May help you get a good night's sleep
- Kills bacteria inside the body as well as outside (apply to wounds for quick healing)

- Helps with diarrhea—especially traveler's diarrhea
- Helps with asthma
- Contributes to strong bones

Pleasant words are as a honeycomb, sweet to the soul, and health to the bones.

Proverbs 16:24 NKJ

Types of Honey

1. *Liquid Honey*: Free of visible crystals, liquid honey is extracted from the honeycomb by centrifugal force, gravity, or straining. Because liquid honey mixes easily into a variety of foods, it's especially convenient for cooking and baking. Most of the honey produced in the United States is sold in the liquid form.

2. *Comb Honey*: Comb honey is honey that comes as it was produced—in the honeybees' wax comb. The comb, as well as the honey, is edible! It may be packaged in several different ways, from small round or square containers to entire frames straight from the hive.

3. *Liquid/Cut Comb Honey*: Cut comb honey is liquid honey that has added chunks of the honeycomb in the jar. This is also known as liquid-cut comb combination.

4. *Naturally Crystallized Honey*: Honey sometimes takes on a semi-solid state that is known as crystallized or granulated honey. This natural phenomenon happens when glucose, one of three main sugars in honey, spontaneously precipitates out of the supersaturated honey solution. The glucose loses water (becoming glucose monohydrate) and takes the form of a crystal (a solid body with a precise and orderly structure). The crystals form a lattice, which immobilizes other components of honey in a suspension, thus creating the semi-solid state.

5. Foodie Tip: If your honey is crystallized, and you prefer to use it as a liquid, simply place the honey jar in warm water and stir until the crystals dissolve. Be careful not to boil or scorch the honey. Also keep in mind that you can eat the honey in a crystallized form. Just scoop it out of the jar and spread it on your toast or drop it in your tea.

6. *Dried Honey*: Dried honey products available commercially for industrial use are derived from pure liquid honey (a) to which processing aids and other ingredients have been added, (b) which have been dried to low moisture content, and (c) which, in most cases, have been converted to a free-flowing product. Dried honey products are available commercially in several forms, including powders, flakes, granules, and crystals. The vast majority of commercial dried honey products are formulated and processed to be free flowing.

Uses of Honey:

1. Beverages – honey works well in coffee and teas. The most suitable is the clover honey but other varieties will sweeten as well.

2. Baking (cakes, muffins, tarts, cookies)—Here are some simple steps to follow when substituting honey for sugar in a recipe;

   - Choose an easy recipe and begin by substituting half the sugar for honey until you have experimented. If it works well then the next time you can increase to a higher percentage of honey.
   - Up to one cup, honey can be substituted for sugar in equal amounts. For example, you can substitute 1/2 cup of honey for 1/2 cup of sugar called for in a recipe. Over one cup, use about 2/3-3/4 cup of honey for every cup of sugar. This is because honey is actually sweeter than sugar.
   - Honey is a liquid, so you'll need to reduce the liquid in the recipe a little. Do this at a rate of 1/4 cup less liquid for every cup of honey used in the recipe.
   - Add ½ teaspoon baking soda for every cup of honey used in a recipe (this is when substituting and not when the original recipe called for it).
   - Honey causes baked goods to brown more quickly, so reduce the oven temperature by 25 degrees Fahrenheit and monitor closely.

3. Meats/Sauces: Honey adds a special flavor to sauces or preparing meats.

4. Toast Spread/Pancakes topping: some of the best syrups are made from a honey base. Check out the *Healthy Treasures* cookbook for some tasty ideas.

5. Anti-diarrhea mixture: Pour 8 ounces of distilled water and ¼ teaspoon of baking soda in a glass. In another glass, mix 8 ounces of orange juice, a pinch of salt, and ½ teaspoon of honey. Alternate drinking from each glass.

6. Sore throats: Folk medicine calls for a gargle of honey mixed with lemon juice or apple cider vinegar. This coats and lubricates the irritated linings of the throat, which makes swallowing easier. On a more scientific level, the ingredient that makes it taste sweet also goes straight to the brain and signals the pituitary gland to start pumping out soothing endorphins.

Foodie tip: Honey has the power to make us feel better by improving our mood, and also think better by stimulating the part of the brain responsible for learning.

Honey Helps during Pregnancy

Heartburn during Pregnancy

Heartburn during pregnancy is one of the most common side-effects of pregnancy. Hormones released during pregnancy allow the softening of the sphincter between the esophagus and stomach. When this happens, stomach acids back up into the esophagus, causing a burning sensation. This may also occur in the latter months of pregnancy as your baby pushes all of your organs upward. You may experience heartburn as a burning sensation in your throat or chest. Other women experience heartburn as a large lump-like feeling in their throat or upper chest. Fortunately, there are ways to minimize your heartburn woes during pregnancy. Mixing some honey with your milk is very good for helping neutralize the excess of stomach acid. Drink a glass of milk every night before going to bed.

Colds during Pregnancy

Colds are quite common during pregnancy. Pregnant women tend to be more susceptible, as their immune systems are lowered and their mucous membranes tend to swell. This can make it more difficult to get rid of coughs and colds, and can make breathing easily a challenge. If you do catch a cold, you can increase your consumption of vitamin C-rich foods, including fruits and fruit juices. Many women find sipping teas, including lemon and honey tea, can help alleviate a sore and uncomfortable throat.

Morning Sickness

Morning sickness is a common experience for pregnant women. About 70% of all women experience nausea and/or vomiting during pregnancy, especially in their first trimester. In more severe cases, morning sickness can also lead to weight loss, malnutrition, or other more serious health complications for the mother and developing child.

Traditional remedies for expectant mothers trying to treat the nausea and vomiting of early pregnancy include soda and crackers, which are only marginally helpful. Ginger is effective against ailments of the reproductive and digestive systems because it stimulates circulation and supports a good blood supply to these organs. Modest amounts of ginger tea with honey are a great remedy for nausea and vomiting. In the early weeks of pregnancy, the further stimulation of blood flow into the abdomen is not recommended, so go easy on ginger at this time.

Caution

While there are many natural remedies during pregnancy, and honey remedies are known to be quite safe in helping to relieve some of the common side effects or complaints of pregnancy (honey is not allowed for newborn and young children under one year old, though), bear in mind that just because something is natural does not always mean it is safe. For instance, there are many herbs that are best avoided during pregnancy. As with anything, during pregnancy, when you are in doubt, always check in with your medical doctor if he or she is educated in nutrition and natural substances.

Is it honey that you have found? Eat what is sufficient for you, that you may not take too much of it and have to vomit it up.

Proverbs 25:16

HEALTHY
SUBSTITUTIONS

NEED AN INGREDIENT for a recipe? What if you are out of an ingredient and in the middle of making dinner? What do you do? What is a healthy substitute for the meal you are making? As you read the substitutions listed below, you will discover new treasures in creating a healthy meal.

Baking powder: use two parts cream of tartar, one part baking soda, and two parts arrowroot.
Bread crumbs: use toasted oats, sesame seeds, cooked brown rice, or other cracked grains.
Butter: in baking, use canola oil, safflower oil, or applesauce (up to ½ cup per recipe). If using butter, use only organic.
Buttermilk: 1 cup = 1 cup minus 1 tablespoon of soy milk, rice milk, or almond milk, plus 1 tablespoon of lemon juice.
Cheese: use equal amounts of soy or almond cheese.
Cheese, cottage cheese: Here is a recipe to make a substitution.

> 1 lbs. Firm tofu, mashed – tofu is a soy product – should state non-GMO on label
>
> 1 TBS Olive oil
>
> 1 TBS Rice or apple-cider vinegar
>
> 2 TBS Lemon juice
>
> ¼ to ½ tsp onion powder, to taste
>
> ¼ to ½ tsp salt or tamari, to taste

Mix half of the tofu and the remaining ingredients in blender. Mix in remaining mashed tofu.
Cheese, cream cheese: You can make your own yo-cheese as a substitute for cream cheese. Your recipes and family will never know the difference, and the health benefits will increase.

Strain yogurt in yogurt strainer, or coffee filter placed in strainer, for 24 hours (set in refrigerator while draining).

Cheese, Ricotta:

>   1 lbs. Firm tofu, mashed

>   ¼ cup olive oil

>   ½ tsp. Nutmeg

>   ½ tsp salt or tamari

Mix half of the tofu and the remaining ingredients in a blender. Mix in remaining tofu.

Chocolate: 1 square or 1 ounce = 3 TBS Carob plus 1 TBS Oil and 1 TBS Water

Cocoa: 1 cup = 1 cup carob powder

Cornstarch: 1 TBS = 1 tablespoon arrowroot powder (Organic non-GMO cornstarch is now available.), tapioca flour can be used as a thickener and is a healthy choice.

Currants: raisins

Flour, white (baking):

>   1 cup = 1 cup corn flour

>   1 cup = ¾ cup coarse cornmeal

>   1 cup = 7/8 cup rice flour

>   1 cup = 1 1/3 cup spelt flour

>   1 cup = 1 cup kamut

>   1 cup = ½ cup barley flour + ¼ cup rice flour + ½ TBS Arrowroot powder

Garlic: 1 clove = 1 tsp minced or ½ tsp powder

Pepper: 1 tsp. Black pepper = ¼ tsp. Cayenne

Sugar, brown:

>   1 cup = ½ cup date sugar and ½ cup honey

>   1 cup = ½ to ¾ cup honey

>   1 cup = ¾ cup maple syrup

Sugar, white:

>   1 cup = 1 cup Fruit Source

>   1 cup = ¾ cup to 1 cup sucanat (honey crystals)

>   1 cup = ¾ cup maple syrup

>   1 cup = ¾ cup honey

>   1 cup = 1 cup rice syrup

>   1 cup = 1 cup molasses, plus ½ tsp baking soda

Worcestershire Sauce: 3 TBS = ¼ cup tamari

Yogurt: equal amount of organic tofu

PART 2: VALUE YOUR VITAMINS

He who has the Son has the life; he who does not have the Son of God does not have the life.

1 John 5:12

Are Vitamins in Scripture?

IN THE EARLY 1900s, nutrients in foods were thought to be *amines* or organic compounds. Since they are vital to life, they were termed "vit-amines," and the first vitamin was produced. Before the 1900s, and even through today, natural vitamins are obtained from the foods God designed to build health.

Today our choices are complicated. We have two problems: the ground has not been managed to contain the highest level of nutrients by rotating crops and letting the field rest every seven years, and we have been genetically modifying the seeds. The bottom line is we are no longer in the Garden of Eden. This means that many of the health problems we are experiencing are due to lack of nutrients. When you understand this, you will need to make a decision as to whether or not to take supplements. Vitamins are not a cure-all or an excuse to eat what you want. Instead, they will only help cure or prevent a disease that is caused by a deficiency of that vitamin. Therefore we need to eat a variety of foods and then consider the need for supplementation.

As you read "These People Don't Need Vitamins," realize that it is almost impossible to get what we need in today's culture. On the pages that follow, are listed reasons for certain nutrients and information on what foods contain the highest level of each nutrient. High-quality food is the best source for valuable vitamins. From this information you can decide if supplements are beneficial. If so, guidelines are listed for quality supplements. We hope you find this information useful.

As far as the question "are supplements in Scripture?" our answer would be a definite maybe. How is that for an answer? The foods containing all natural vitamins are definitely in Scripture, but the isolated nutrients are not.

Check out the next few pages, and read the checklist for high-quality supplements. Remember, the most expensive vitamin you can take is one that does not work or contributes free radicals from the chemicals included.

These People Don't Need Vitamins

If you meet these criteria, then you don't need to take vitamin supplements:

- Eat a high-quality protein that contains all nine essential amino acids daily.
- Drink 6–8 cups of purified water daily.
- Eat a minimum of 10–12 servings of fresh fruits and veggies daily.
- Eat a diet of 50% raw veggies and fruits daily and organic always.
- Do not eat processed, refined, pre-packaged, or instant foods.
- Refrain from all junk foods, white flour, hydrogenated oils, trans fats, and fast food.
- Do not consume caffeine, alcohol, cigarettes, drugs, medications, etc.
- Have at least two bowel movements daily.
- Exercise daily.
- Do not put any chemicals/toxins in your body (foods or drinks containing pesticides, herbicides, hormones, antibiotics, flavorings, colorings, preservatives, etc.).
- Do not put any chemicals/toxins on your body (cosmetics, personal care products, chlorine, laundry and cleaning products residues, etc.).
- Do not breathe in any chemicals/toxins (outdoor pollution, indoor pollution from cleaning or personal care products, off-gassing of carpets, paints, construction materials, etc.).
- You have a healthy family history.
- You do not suffer from any conditions, illnesses, headaches, or health challenges.
- You live a relaxed, stress-free, positive, happy life.

Congratulations if you are one of these people!

Why Do We Need to Supplement?

The information in this book along with the recipes in the *Healthy Treasures Cookbook* are a great place to initiate building health, but without supplementing, you may still be missing some vital nutrients necessary to rebuild healthy cells. Your body is building one trillion cells each day with the recipe of nutrients we give it, so let's improve the ingredients available to make a great recipe! As you look for a high-quality whole food supplement (foodlet) and continue taking it for a minimum of three months or up to a year, you will see great benefits in how you feel.

A study published in the *Nutrition Journal*, October 2007, proved the value of taking supplements and even multiple supplements. You can research this study by going to www.landmarkstudy.com. There you will read the study which evaluated people who took several high quality supplements for over 20 years verses people who took only one multivitamin verses those who took none at all. All this data was compared using the NHANES data base and coordinated by Gladys Block, PhD University of California, Berkeley. It is worth the time to research this study to completely understand how supplements make a vital difference.

> It is the paradox of modern man to supplement his diet or suffer with chronic degenerative disease.
>
> ~Dr. Roger Williams

Four Reasons for Supplements

- *Restoration*—following downturns in health due to nutrient deficiency.
- *Repair*—following injury to tissues such as surgery, chemo-therapies, affects of chemicals, sports injuries, etc.
- *Resist*—further damage due to daily stresses.
- *Maintenance and to achieve optimal health*—daily intake of key nutrients will help us maintain the health we have acquired through healthy eating, while increasing our intake will help us reach the optimal health level.

NOTE: Each person is unique, and no two days have the same requirements.

Many doctors and scientist have known for years that supplements are necessary to obtain optimal health. It is difficult to acquire the amount of nutrients in our daily diet. The Journal of the American Medical Association, June 19, 2002, stated, "…the use of vitamin supplements is a prudent intervention in the fight against many chronic degenerative diseases… Sub-optimal intake of some vitamins, even above levels causing classic vitamin deficiency, is a risk factor for chronic diseases."[39, 40]

> The next major advance in the health of the American people will be determined by what the individual is willing to do for himself.
>
> ~John Knowles

"Vitamins" and "Minerals"—Definitions

There is a lot of confusion regarding the definition of these words. This section will increase your understanding of their meanings and your need for both.

Vitamins:

- Are essential* to life.
- Regulate metabolism.
- Assist the biochemical processes that releases energy from digested food.
- Work with enzymes as coenzymes, which enable the body to perform its activities, such as building and feeding cells.

* *Essential* means that it must be acquired by diet or supplements; your body cannot manufacture it.

Minerals:

- Are needed for proper composition of body fluids.
- Are necessary for the formation of blood and bone.
- Maintain healthy nerve function.
- Function as coenzymes.
- Enable the body to perform its activities; they build and feed cells.
- Are needed in varying amounts and are co-factors crucial to the body's health.
- Include:
  - Boron
  - Calcium
  - Chromium
  - Cobalt
  - Copper
  - Iodine
  - Iron
  - Magnesium
  - Manganese
  - Molybdenum
  - Phosphorus
  - Potassium
  - Selenium
  - Silicon
  - Sodium
  - Sulfur

- Vanadium
- Zinc
- Plus numerous others in varied trace amounts.

Fat-Soluble Vitamins:
- A, D, E, and K
- Require the presence of fatty acids (EFA) to be transported and absorbed. Fat-free diets, therefore, interfere with their absorption, creating possible deficiencies.
- Are transported directly through the lymph system first, then through the blood stream.
- Are stored in body tissues. They can be eaten in large amounts once in a while and still meet the body's need over time.

Water-Soluble Vitamins:
- B and C*
- Are not stored in the body; therefore, they are quickly depleted.
- Are retained for varying periods in the body. A single day's omission does not bring on a deficiency, but still they must be eaten or supplemented regularly.
- Must be regularly consumed/replenished.
- Should be taken in divided doses throughout the day.
- Are absorbed directly into the blood stream.

*We must obtain vitamin C from our diets, as humans cannot manufacture it.

Enzymes: Enzymes are protein chemicals that carry a vital energy feature needed for every chemical action and reaction that occurs in our bodies. There are approximately 20,000 different enzymes found in the human cell. These enzymes combine with co-enzymes (vitamins and minerals) to form nearly 100,000 chemical reactions each second of your life. These reactions enable us to see, hear, feel, move, digest food, and think.

Co-enzymes: Vitamins and minerals are co-enzymes. A co-enzyme is dependent on the energy from an enzyme. It combines to form another enzyme. Vitamin C is a co-enzyme that combines with an enzyme for collagen production.

Bioavailability: refers to the rate at which an element enters the blood stream and is utilized by specific organs or tissues. This is dependent on several factors, such as the:

- Efficiency of digestion and time of transit through the digestive system.
- Previous nutrient intake and nutrition status.

- Other foods consumed at the same time.
- Method of preparation—raw, cooked, or processed.
- Source of the nutrient (synthetic, fortified, or naturally occurring).

Organic and Natural: Understanding These Terms
Regarding Supplementation

There is no legal definition of "natural," and until October, 2002, there was no legal definition for the term "organic." Hence, the terms have long been used in marketing to convey a general sense of purity and wholesomeness, but without specific meaning. The USDA has outlined how foods labeled "organic" must be produced and handled, and these standards took effect on October 21, 2002. Products labeled as "organic" now need to meet one of three standards:

1. Produce that has been exclusively cultivated and processed according to the new organic standards is permitted to bear the USDA "100% Organic" seal.
2. Packaged goods in which 95% of the ingredients by weight have been organically produced can be labeled "Organic."
3. Packaged goods with 70 to 95% organic ingredients by weight may be labeled "Made with Organic," and the specific organic ingredients need to be listed.

Products made with less than 70% organic ingredients are permitted only to list organic ingredients in the ingredient panel and cannot use the word "organic" in primary labeling.

For the record, "*organic*," while worthwhile, *does not ensure purity or potency*. And due to the multi-sourced nature of food and nutritional supplements, applying the term under the new standards is not workable in many cases. This is because many raw ingredients are grown in the wild, not on organic farms. Such ingredients are not eligible to bear the "organic" label. Additionally, the organic standard applies only in the US. Many botanical ingredients are sourced from other countries and, therefore, are not eligible to bear the "organic" label.

As far as "*natural*" is concerned, it *has no legal definition*. Anything not fresh off the plant, tree, or vine is less than natural—something must happen between the time raw ingredients are harvested and when they are formulated into an end product. A good working definition of "natural" would be, "as close to nature as possible, with the least amount of processing needed to deliver claimed nutrients."

When comparing supplement companies, the words "natural" and "organic" may not be found on the label since these words, as mentioned above, have no meaning. Instead, look for peer-reviewed research. Make sure the company is using the finest natural sources for its formulations and that they use pure, highly bio-available nutrients from nature and natural resources.

WHO'S TESTING YOUR SUPPLEMENTS?

BY STEPHEN G. CHANEY, PH.D.

IT'S RELIABLE TO continue getting your supplements from a company that you know and trust, a company that does clinical studies on their products and performs rigorous quality controls. You know their products are pure, safe and effective.

Then one day you're shopping in your favorite drug store or discount store and you see the same supplements for just a couple of dollars.

You can't help thinking, "Wow! Here's the same stuff I've been taking for a lot less money! Why not save my money?" you reason. "Is it possible that they have run some quality control tests on their products? After all, how bad can they be?" The truth is that the answer to this sort of reasoning lies in the fact that these products are of inferior quality.

The events on March 2, 2010 illustrate just how bad. On this date the makers and sellers of fish oil supplements were sued by the Mateel Environmental Justice Foundation in California for not telling consumers that their products contained toxic levels of PCBs.

I find it amusing and somewhat scary that the FDA did not initiate this action and force the manufacturers to take their contaminated products off the shelves. Instead an environmental consumers group had to sue them for not including PCBs on the label! They sued them under California proposition 65 which requires a warning label whenever a product contains toxic ingredients.

The defendants in this lawsuit were Omega Protein, a Houston-based company that is the world's largest producer of omega-3 fish oil, and the many companies that they produced fish oil for - companies like Rite Aid, CVS, GNC, Now Health Group, Pharmavite, Solgar and Twinlab.

And those aren't the only ones. The Mateel Environmental Justice Foundation only tested 10 omega-3 supplements manufactured by Omega Protein to date and have found PCBs in all of them. They plan to continue testing and to add other companies to the lawsuit if their products are also contaminated.

Even scarier is that many of labels on these products said that the omega-3 supplement was treated to reduce or remove PCBs. As a consumer you were led to believe that they were safe! The bottom line is that the manufacturer probably didn't test for PCBs and neither did the companies selling their omega-3 supplements to the consumer. The alternative - that they tested the products, knew that they were contaminated with PCBs and sold them to the public anyway - is even worse.

As if that weren't scary enough the FDA announced a massive recall of products containing textured vegetable protein manufactured by a company called Basic Food Flavors because of salmonella contamination. The problem is that there are at least 56 different kinds of consumer products containing this company's textured vegetable protein - including salad dressings, dips, packaged snacks, potato chips and soup mixes (Who knew that salad dressings contained textured vegetable protein?).

That means that this recall will be huge. It will affect many foods that most people buy and use every day. Once again, the problem is that neither the manufacturer nor the companies using the textured vegetable protein had run the basic quality control assays that would have detected salmonella contamination.

So what can you do as a consumer? Here are my recommendations:

1) Get your supplements from an established company with a reputation for quality and integrity. I would recommend choosing a company that has been around for a number of years so that you know that their reputation is based on their track record over the years rather than just on hype.

2) Make sure that they run rigorous quality controls on their products. I would choose a company that requires pharmaceutical grade quality controls on their products.

3) Make sure that they have published clinical studies on their products that prove both safety and effectiveness. Again I would recommend choosing a company that has many published clinical studies on their products rather than just one or two.

CONSUMER CHECKLIST FOR HIGH-QUALITY VITAMIN SUPPLEMENTS

1. *Do you have a way to tell if the supplement (vitamin) that you're using is being absorbed and assimilated?* The place to begin is to see if your supplement dissolves within 30 minutes or less when placed in water. That is the same standard the pharmaceutical industry uses for tablets. Otherwise, your supplement goes in one end and out the other.

2. *Are the supplements you are taking being absorbed and assimilated into the bloodstream where they are available to the cells?* Always ask the company for peer reviewed research on its products. The key word here is *peer reviewed*. That means it is unbiased,

legitimate research instead of advertising research, where you pay someone to publish your research in what looks like a legitimate journal. If the company does not have peer-reviewed research, then shop elsewhere. You want proof!

3. *Is there balance in the formulation?* Balance is critical to a well-formulated supplement. Many nutrients do not work effectively unless they are in a certain balance. For example, The B vitamin Biotin is extremely expensive. It should offer at least 100% of the daily value. Most vitamins will show none at all or less than 100%. That is a sign to you of a poorly formulated vitamin, so read your labels.

4. *Is the amount on the label the amount in each tablet?* A common problem in the food supplement industry is quality control. It is not uncommon for the amount in each individual tablet in a bottle of supplements to vary dramatically. Ask the company for proof that their products contain all the ingredients listed on the label.

5. *Is the manufacturer using a "cooling" system to preserve nutrients?* When supplements are manufactured at a low temperature, all the vitamins, minerals, enzymes, and phytonutrients are not lost in the process. Without the enzymes, the body cannot utilize or absorb the nutrients effectively. It is common for companies to use too much heat and pressure in making their tablets, which destroys the enzymes.

6. *Are sugars, artificial colorings, or sweeteners used?* It is common for vitamins to have artificial coloring and sweeteners in them. Read the labels to determine their presence.

7. *Are the supplements you are using safe, and do you trust the company to have your best interest in mind over profit?* You can get this answer as you investigate the company's history and long-term studies. Don't buy a product just because you like the sales person.

FOUNDATION IS A MULTIVITAMIN

The base of any supplement program is a multivitamin with minerals, containing at least 400 micrograms (0.4 milligrams) of the B vitamin folic acid. Multivitamins are the most commonly used product in the dietary supplement category. There are thirteen recognized vitamins, and products called "multivitamins" must have all of them in addition to an assortment of minerals. There are twelve minerals for which "reference daily intakes" have been established by the Food and Drug Administration, for purposes of nutrition labeling.

ALFALFA

Alfalfa is no longer for just horses. The supplemental alfalfa has tremendous healing and prevention abilities.

Questions you need to ask:

- Does your family's antiperspirant seem to be doing the job? How about their foot spray or powder?
- Is this allergy season affecting you or your family?
- What about this summer heat? Do your ankles swell?
- Do you ever find it hard to take off your rings?

Do you know the benefits of alfalfa?

- Loaded with chlorophyll, a natural body deodorizer. If you were to use an analogy for alfalfa's function, it is like building a healthy body house and alfalfa is the window—you open it to give you fresh, clean air.
- Loaded with trace minerals. Trace minerals balance salt levels. Salt controls fluid retention, and fluid retention plays a big role in inflammation and pain.
- Beneficial in reducing inflammation. It is helpful for cystitis or inflammation of the bladder, provides relief from bloating or water retention (especially during PMS), and aids the reduction of the swelling and inflammation of arthritis. Any nerve damage (temporary) sees an increase in fluid to the injured area—more fluid retention means more swelling. Alfalfa reduces the swelling.
- Helpful to babies born by C-section who are loaded with mucus because they haven't gone through the birth canal. Air connects with the mucous in the lungs and nose, and it thickens. These babies have harder time breathing when lying down. Giving Alfalfa tea can help make the mucous soluble, and after a few days, they can sneeze and cough it up.
- Awesome in controlling allergy symptoms while helping a person to rebuild an overactive immune system.
- Loaded with enzymes, helps with digestion, and helps nursing moms who are having a hard time producing enough milk to produce more.

Alfalfa has been used for centuries, since it was first discovered by the Arabs. The leaves of the plant are rich in minerals, nutrients, vitamins, fiber, and protein. The roots grow deep into the soil, sometimes as much as 130 feet. This allows the plants to pull in the rich minerals that are deep in the soil. A good supplement would use a plant that has roots growing at least twenty-five feet into the soil.

In 1597, English herbalist John Gerard recommended alfalfa for upset stomachs. Later, noted biologist Frank Bouer discovered that the leaves of this remarkable legume contain eight essential amino acids. And we now know that the plant contains three components that appear to have special functions: bioflavonoids, dietary fiber, and trace minerals.

Bioflavonoids

According to the research work of Elliot Middleton, Jr. M.D., certain bioflavonoids found in alfalfa may play a role in allergic reactions. They may inhibit the release of histamine from white blood cells. They also possibly may serve as an anti-inflammatory agent. Many types of arthritis, such as rheumatoid arthritis, are believed to be auto-immune diseases in which the body releases histamine as a response to a perceived "invasion." If histamine is blocked, inflammation may subside.

Specialized Fiber

Alfalfa may be one of the most effective fiber sources when dried; it contains 22% fiber. It has been observed that it has the ability to inhibit the buildup of cholesterol.

Other interesting studies done by Dr. Benjamin Erschoff showed protective effects from toxins. He fed a group of rats a pure diet, and they gained weight. Then he added a toxin, Red Dye #2, to their diet. Growth stopped. They became sick and died within two weeks. A similar group of rats were fed the same toxic diet with 10% alfalfa meal added. The toxins were neutralized, and the rats gained weight.

But the protective effect is greater than just fiber. One theory is the saponins (gum-like plant substances) in alfalfa give the fiber its binding capabilities. Another source of saponins is legumes, especially soybeans, noted for lowering cholesterol. Alfalfa possesses tremendous binding capabilities. It also has been hypothesized that alfalfa fiber binds with antigens that cause antibody reactions, many entering from the nasal passages. Alfalfa might help eliminate these irritations.

Trace Minerals

Alfalfa is very rich in a wide variety of trace minerals: calcium, phosphorous, magnesium, iron, copper, zinc, and iodine. There are also trace amounts of chromium, molybdenum, selenium, manganese, tin, and nickel.

Alfalfa may be used to relieve:
- Allergies.
- Anemia.
- Any inflammatory problem.
- Arthritis.
- Athlete's foot.
- Bleeding gums. Vitamin C works for this also.
- Body and breath odor.

- Cystitis, or inflammation of the bladder.
- Gout.
- Headaches, including migraines.
- Lowers cholesterol
- Poor digestion or bowel problems.
- Sinus problems.
- Toxins in the body.
- Water retention.

Alfalfa is a good laxative and a natural diuretic. It is often used to treat urinary tract infections. This versatile herb is also a traditional remedy for arthritis and is reputed to be an excellent overall tonic.

Although mostly sold in tablets, alfalfa sprouts are especially effective. When using sprouts, be sure and clean well with Basic H2[41] to remove all mold and bacteria.

When made into a tea, alfalfa can be given to babies to help with sinus drainage and colds. Be careful only to use supplements from a reputable source with studies to ensure quality, potency, and purity.

People who have been diagnosed with any auto-immune disorder should avoid alfalfa seeds or sprouts. Pure, uncontaminated leaves, as in a supplement, however, may be beneficial to those with auto-immune disorders.

CAUTION: Alfalfa is now being grown in areas of the country as a GMO crop. When purchasing alfalfa do your research to make sure it is from a trusted source.

VITAMIN A AND BETA-CAROTENE

Vitamin A, also called retinol, and Beta-carotene have become very popular and yet are still somewhat confusing. Let's look at the basic information to understand the need for them in your diet.

Benefits of Vitamin A and Beta-carotene:
Vitamin A may be the most versatile of the fat-soluble vitamins because of its role in several important body processes. Its role in promoting good night vision, the health of mucous membranes and skin, and the growth of the body's tissues are well documented by research. The following are some other roles that vitamin A plays in the body. Vitamin A:

- Aids in utilizing protein.
- Helps heal skin lesions, cuts, and wounds.
- Helps the adrenal gland (hormones).

- Helps the thyroid gland (hormones).
- Improves immunity—protects against colds, flu, and infections.
- Is necessary for growth of bones, testicular function, ovarian function, embryonic development, and regulation of growth.
- Is necessary for new cell growth, nerve cell sheaths, and red blood cells.
- Is vital to the thymus gland
- May inhibit certain types of cancers.
- Mucosal integrity.
- Plays a vital role in vision – protects against macular degeneration.
- Plays an important role in fighting infection—prevents invasion of bacteria and viruses.
- Protects against cataract formation.
- Slows the aging process.
- Speeds healing, especially after surgery, severe burns, or injuries.

Vitamin A is found in foods of animal origin (meats, eggs, fish, dairy). Beta-carotene, also known as pro-vitamin A, is found in the pigments of fruits and veggies. It is a precursor to vitamin A, meaning the body can convert beta-carotene into vitamin A when it is needed. Your intestinal enzymes make this conversion during the digestive process. Any excess dietary intake of beta-carotene is deposited into fatty tissues throughout the body until it is required for conversion into vitamin A. Beta-carotene is a safe way to ensuring optimal vitamin A levels, as it is non-toxic even in larger amounts. Beta-carotene is also the best source of vitamin A because it is converted in the liver into only the amount of vitamin A that the body actually needs. Vitamin A taken as a supplement (especially in a synthetic form) may be toxic to the liver in large amounts.

If you are pregnant, do not take more than 10,000 IU of vitamin A daily because of reported birth development problems. Beta-carotene is safe during pregnancy.

Note that antibiotics, laxatives, and some cholesterol-lowering drugs interfere with the absorption of vitamin A.

Foods that are natural sources for Vitamin A and Beta-carotene:
- Alfalfa
- Apricots, fresh
- Asparagus
- Broccoli
- Cantaloupe
- Carrots
- Cayenne
- Eggs

- Endive, raw
- Kale
- Leaf Lettuce
- Mustard Greens
- Papayas
- Paprika
- Peaches
- Pumpkin
- Red Clover
- Red Peppers
- Sage
- Salmon
- Spinach
- Squash, Winter
- Sweet Potatoes
- Tomatoes
- Watermelon

Those consuming a varied diet rich in green vegetables and carrots ensure efficient sources for meeting vitamin A needs. Vitamin A and beta-carotene can be destroyed by heat; light and by air. Carrot juice is rich in this substance only if it is consumed directly after pressings.[41]

Signs of Vitamin A Deficiency*: Can be caused by alcohol, digestive problems, and inadequate diets.

- Dry hair and/or skin
- Dryness of the conjunctiva or cornea (lack of tear production)
- Poor growth or growth retardation
- Night blindness—one of the first detectable signs of vitamin A deficiency
- Abscesses in the ears
- Insomnia
- Fatigue
- Reproductive difficulties
- Sinusitis
- Pneumonia
- Frequent colds
- Respiratory infections
- Skin disorders, including acne

- Weight loss
- Poor bone growth
- Weak tooth enamel

*Note that deficiency symptoms usually occur together with protein and zinc deficiencies.

What to look for in a supplement:
- Should be in a liquid form. The nutrients are inert in a dry form.
- Should be separate from the multi-vitamin but not replace a multi-vitamin
- Should contain at least five key carotenoids(there are over 400 now known) and three other phytonutrients:
  - Beta carotene—beneficial for the cervix, prostate, eyes, lungs, and heart
  - Alpha carotene
  - Lycopene—most potent of all carotenes and may help everyone in
  - lowering cancer risk
  - Lutein—closely related to zeaxanthin; concentrates in the retina
  - Zeaxanthin—may help prevent macular degeneration
  - Quercetin—may help with lung cancer
  - Grapeseed extract—helps with the small vessels in the body (veins, capillaries)
  - Sulforaphane—protects cells against toxic chemicals
- The label (or literature) must state how many servings of each fruit, veggie, and fish are guaranteed to be in each serving of the supplement.
- The manufacturer must conduct at least 200–300 tests for contaminants, including lead, fungicides, and harmful solvents. Contaminants in our foods supply contribute to health problems. So we don't want them in the supplement.
- Studies to prove the supplement works are peer-reviewed, double blind studies.

Note that fast foods often lack vitamin A. Anyone who dines frequently on hamburgers, French fries, and colas would be wise to emphasize colorful vegetables and fruits at other meals.

B-COMPLEX

B vitamins are well thought of as "the energy pill" and also the "nerve supplement". Though they actually do not give energy to the body, they do, in fact, serve as helpers to the enzymes that release energy from carbohydrates, fats, and protein. It is true that without B vitamins our bodies would lack energy.

There are Eight B vitamins that make up the B-Complex:

B1—Thiamine - Low amounts connected with diabetes

B2—Riboflavin – good for energizing cells

B3—Niacin – works to inactivate hormones

B5—Pantothenic acid – comes in all whole foods

B6—Pyridoxine – helps with nerves, low levels seen in ADD/ADHD, blocks herbicides from being absorbed

B12—Cobalamin – prevents senility

Biotin – improves glucose metabolism, alopecia, hair health, comes from food and is produced in a healthy gut

Folic Acid - low amounts of folate (folic acid) are shown in breast cancer

Why Do I Need B Vitamins?

- They are water-soluble; therefore, any excess is excreted and not stored by the body. They must be continually replaced.
- Stress depletes supplies of B.
- Sulfa drugs, sleeping pills, insecticides, and estrogen deplete B vitamins.
- Our processed diet, including sugar and alcohol, plays a major role in depleting B-Complex from the body.
- Remember: no B, no energy!

How Do I Take B-Complex?

The most important thing to remember is that all the B vitamins should be taken together when possible. They are so interrelated in function that large doses of any of them may be therapeutically valueless or may cause a deficiency of others. B vitamins work together in the body and many of them are found in the same foods.

In nature, the B-complex vitamins are found in:

- Yeast
- Green vegetables
- Whole grains
- Eggs
- Salmon

Nowhere in nature is there a single B vitamin isolated from the rest. Most preparations of single B vitamins are synthetic or at least no longer in their natural form. The balance or amount of each B vitamin is already set by God, and that is how it is in natural food sources or whole food supplements. If the balance is off, too much of one B vitamin can throw your body's ability to utilize the others properly. A deficiency in one often indicates a deficiency in another.

Biotin and folic acid are the most expensive B vitamins. Biotin is about eighteen times as costly as silver and takes approximately three months to produce. If you are purchasing a B-complex vitamin, make sure it has at least the 100% RDA for each of these vitamins. Some studies show that 100 milligrams daily can decrease the chance of hair loss in men.

New studies have proven that time-released B vitamins, together with a time-released vitamin C, will give you a steadier dose of B vitamins and fewer supplements may be required to achieve the desired effect. Most time-released B-Complex supplements have not been proven to work, as the balance is difficult to achieve.

The absorption of B-Complex may be compromised if a person has been taking antibiotics as a medication or in his or her foods (beef, chicken, and dairy products). For this reason, a person may want to make sure he or she is eating a high-quality yogurt or taking probiotics.

Roles of B-Complex:

1. It enables the body to release energy from food. If the food you eat has been deprived of the B vitamins, you are asking your body to burn sugar, flour, etc., without "wicks." The results will be lack of energy, tiredness, indigestion, and constipation.

2. B vitamins enhance the nervous system. They are necessary for proper nerve transmission. They are important for mental and emotional stability. Signs of deficiencies in this area are mood swings, depression, nervousness, hyperactivity, schizophrenia, and irritability.

3. Stress plays a major role in depleting these vitamins. Your adrenal gland depends on the B vitamins to work properly, enabling you to handle stress in a healthy way.

4. B vitamins are necessary for the proper amount of hormones. PMS, menopause, diabetes, etc., all depend on your body's utilization of these vitamins.

5. B-Complex supports and elevates the metabolism levels.

6. B-Complex is necessary for the formation of protective antibodies, healthy red blood cells, and normal growth. They also contribute to healthy skin, hair, eyes, liver, mouth, digestive tract, muscles, immune system, and proper brain function.

Signs of B-complex deficiencies:
*   abnormal heart rhythms
*   anemia
*   carpal tunnel syndrome
*   confusion
*   constipation

- craving for sweets
- depression
- high cholesterol
- inflammatory bowel
- insomnia
- mouth sores
- numbness in hands and feet
- poor appetite
- poor coordination

These people need extra B-Complex:
- Anyone doing strenuous exercise
- Anyone taking a baby aspirin
- Anyone taking antibiotics
- Babies with cradle cap (biotin)
- Eating a processed food diet
- Smokers
- Those consuming alcohol
- Those on oral birth control pills

These vitamins are found in every cell and must be present continuously for the cells to function as they should. And remember, these are the B-Happy vitamins!

Vitamin C

Two hundred and fifty years ago, any man who joined the crew of a seagoing ship knew he had, at best, a 50/50 chance of returning alive—not because he might be slain by pirates or die in a storm, but because he might contract the dreaded disease called "scurvy." Scurvy is a vitamin C deficiency disease. Sailors would contract the disease after traveling many months on the seas. A British physician found that sailors with scurvy who were given citrus fruits were cured within a short time. The British Navy made use of this information and required all navy vessels to provide lime juice to every sailor daily. The term "limey" was then applied to the British sailors. The name later given to the vitamin, ascorbic acid, means "no scurvy."

Vitamin C is a water-soluble vitamin that must be obtained through the diet or in the form of supplements. It is the only supplement that can be absorbed throughout the entire intestinal tract. A sustained release formula is best, allowing availability throughout the body for longer periods of time.

Vitamin C is very fragile, easily destroyed, and is not stored in the body. Supplements should state they contain bioflavonoids, which means that the manufacturer has included other ingredients that were in the fruit in the supplement. These phytonutrients are necessary for proper assimilation of the vitamin in your body. Some time-released products typically use synthetic binders (plastic release systems) that bind with the nutrients for slow release. Many of these products never break down to be absorbed in the blood stream. Other products use mineral ascorbates with the isolated ascorbic acid to act as a buffering agent. It is essential to use an all-natural, whole-food-based supplement without synthetic ingredients.

Note that vitamin C's potency can be lost through exposure to light, heat, and air. In food preparation, when possible, wait until right before serving to cut, peel, or slice the fruit (organic is best).

Functions of Vitamin C—Two Primary Roles

As a cofactor in collagen formation, vitamin C:

- Helps to form the fibrous structural protein of connective tissues known as collagen. This protein is necessary for the formation of connective tissue in skin, ligaments, teeth, and bones.
- Plays an important role in healing wounds and burns. It is necessary for tissue growth and repair. It also protects against blood clotting and bruising.
- Is necessary for healthy gums.
- Aids in the production of anti-stress hormones and is very important for proper functioning of the adrenal glands.
- Protects against the harmful effects of pollution.
- Helps to prevent cancer.
- Protects against infection and enhances the immune system.
- Increases absorption of iron.
- Strengthens collagen production
- Reduces inflammation

Strong capillaries are dependent on Vitamin C. Nosebleeds, varicose veins, and bruising are all signs of needed Vitamin C.

As an antioxidant, vitamin C:

- Contributes to a healthy heart by reducing cholesterol levels and high blood pressure.
- Fights bacterial infections and reduces the effects on the body of allergy-producing substances. It is great for treating the common cold, allergies, asthma, bronchitis, etc.

- Acts as an antihistamine, decongestant, and anti-inflammatory.
- Is important for the absorption of iron.
- Is a major antioxidant—works well at re-energizing vitamin E.

Signs of Deficiency:
- Allergies
- Bleeding or swollen gums
- Bronchial infections
- Bruising easily
- Cuticles tearing and hangnails
- Edema
- Excessive hair loss
- Frequent colds or flu
- Joint pains
- Muscle weakness
- Nose bleeds
- Poor digestion
- Slow healing of wounds (cuts, scrapes, etc.)
- Stressful life
- Tiredness.
- Varicose veins or broken capillaries

Food Sources:
- Asparagus
- Avocados
- Berries
- Black currants
- Broccoli
- Brussels sprouts
- Cantaloupe
- Citrus fruits (oranges, lemons, grapefruit, etc.)
- Green vegetables – including peas and peppers
- Greens – collards, dandelion greens, kale, spinach, Swiss chard, watercress, mustard greens, beet greens
- Mangoes
- Onions
- Papayas

- Persimmons
- Pineapple
- Radishes
- Rose hips, tomatoes, turnips, and alfalfa.

Interesting Facts

Dr. Frederick R. Kenner used Vitamin C[42] aggressively to cure many diseases, such as chicken pox, measles, mumps, tetanus, and polio, before vaccinations were available. The following is a list of conditions that Dr. Kenner successfully treated with aggressive Vitamin C therapy:

Alcoholism	Arthritis
Atherosclerosis	Bladder infection
Burns and secondary Infections	Chronic Fatigue
Complications of surgery	Corneal Ulcer
Diabetes	Glaucoma
Heat Stroke	Heavy Metal Poisoning (Mercury, Lead)
High cholesterol	Leukemia
Multiple Sclerosis	Radiation Burns
Rocky Mountain Fever	Ruptured Intervertebral Disc
Schizophrenia	Some cancers
Venomous Bites (insects, snakes)	

Because of vitamin C's antioxidant property, food manufacturers sometimes add a synthetic variation of vitamin C to processed foods, including beverages and meat.

CALCIUM

Calcium holds the honor of being the most abundant mineral in the body. Its importance is gaining recognition, as evidenced by magazine articles on osteoporosis.

Calcium is necessary for:

- Formation of strong bones and teeth. Osteoporosis is the twelfth leading cause of death in the US. Bones are constantly being broken down and formed again. In an adult, 20% of bone calcium is reabsorbed (withdrawn from bones) and replaced each year; therefore, every five years bones are renewed.
- Normal cell functioning. If there is not enough calcium in the soft tissue of the body

and fluids surrounding our cells, our bodies will "leach" calcium from their own bones.

- Healthy Gums. Vitamin C is critical as well.
- Regular heartbeat and transmission of nerve impulses.
- Muscle contraction and relaxation. Muscle cramping is a sign of calcium deficiency. PMS and cramping are also a sign of a deficiency of calcium.
- Lowering of blood pressure.
- Blood clotting and helping to prevent cancer.
- Protection against the development of pre-eclampsia during pregnancy.
- Activating several digestive enzymes. It also plays a part in the acid/alkaline balance in your body.
- Is also a natural tranquilizer.

Calcium deficiency can lead to the following problems:

Aching joints,	Brittle nails,
Eczema,	Elevated blood cholesterol,
Heart palpitations,	Hypertension,
Insomnia,	Muscle cramps,
Nervousness,	Numbness in the arms and legs,
Pasty complexion,	Rheumatoid arthritis,
Rickets,	Tooth decay.

Deficiencies can also be associated with cognitive impairment, convulsions, depression, delusions, and hyperactivity.

CALCIUM RICH FOODS

Osteoporosis and bone disease plague all ages in America. Much of this comes from a lack of minerals, such as calcium, in our diets. Minerals in our diet can make a great impact on our health, and it helps to know what foods contribute a healthy quantity.

There are many good sources of dietary minerals. Yogurt is one of the most easily digestible. One cup of yogurt contains about 300 milligrams of calcium. However, a 3.5 ounce can of sardines also contain 300 milligrams of calcium and is loaded with health-enhancing omega-3 fats. Here is a list of foods to add to your bone-building grocery list:

FOOD	AMOUNT	CALCIUM (MG)
Green leafy veggies (cooked, unless otherwise specified)		
collard greens	1 cup	300
wild greens (lambs, quarters, wild onions)	1 cup	350
broccoli	1 cup	150
kale	1 cup	179
spinach	1 cup	278
turnip greens	1 cup	229
beet greens	1 cup	165
bok choy	1 cup	200
mustard greens	1 cup	150
rhubarb	1 cup	348
watercress	1 cup	53
parsley (raw)	1 cup	122
dandelion greens	1 cup	147
Sea veggies (cooked, unless otherwise specified)		
Hijiki	1 cup	610
Wakame	1 cup	520
Kelp	1 cup	305
Agar-agar (used as a thickener)	1 cup	400
Dulse	1 cup (dry)	567
Fish (bones: the major source of calcium in fish)		
Sardines (with bones)	3.5 ounce can, drained	300
Beans and Legumes		
Tofu, firm	4 ounce	80–150
Tempeh	4 ounce	172
Garbanzo beans (chick peas)	1 cup (cooked)	135
Black beans	1 cup (cooked)	135
Pinto beans	1 cup (cooked)	128
Nuts and Seeds		
Sesame seeds (must be ground for absorption)	3 TBSP	300

Almonds	1 cup	300
Sunflower Seeds	1 cup	174
Brazil nuts	1 cup	260
Hazelnuts	1 cup	282

Other sources

Tortillas, corn	2	120
Blackstrap molasses	1 TBSP	137

Dairy

Skim milk	1 cup	300
Whole milk	1 cup	288
Cheese (Swiss, cheddar)	1.5 ounce	300
Ice milk	1 cup	204
Nonfat yogurt	1 cup	294
Cottage cheese (low fat)	1 cup	150

Choosing a calcium supplement:

- Calcium will be better absorbed and utilized by your body if there is adequate magnesium, boron, vitamin K, trace minerals, and vitamin D in the same supplement. Look for a supplement that contains all of these in one tablet. Those with just calcium alone can be more harmful because of the lack of absorption; therefore, your body has to pull calcium from your bones.
- This is a mineral that is better in powder form (tablet), not liquid form.
- Do a disintegration test on your calcium supplements. Place them in water and vinegar. A supplement should dissolve within thirty minutes. There are many supplements that make it whole to your septic tank.
- Be careful with supplements that contain more than 500 milligrams in one tablet. Calcium is a bulky mineral, and a manufacturer would have to compress the tablet too tightly to get that amount in one tablet. They do this to enable you to be able to swallow it. However, it most likely will not breakdown (disintegrate) in your body. It is better to take several tablets.
- Check the tablet coating. Your digestive juices were not made to break through shellac.
- Choose a calcium supplement that does not include bone meal, oyster shell, coral, or dolomite as ingredients. These calcium sources may be contaminated with lead and other heavy metals that are harmful.

- There should be no flavorings, sweeteners, preservatives, or colorings.
- Good choices of calcium would include calcium carbonate, di-calcium phosphate, and citrate.
- Be careful when taking some antacids, as they may actually inhibit the absorption of calcium.

Calcium Absorption

These factors can **decrease** the absorption of calcium:

- Low levels of vitamin D
- Consuming high fiber at the same time
- Decreased need in the body.
- Aging
- Lack of exercise

These factors may **increase** the absorption of calcium

- Increased Vitamin d
- Consuming dairy at the same meal
- Increased need such as growth, pregnancy, lactation
- Parathyroid hormone
- Lack of stress
- Digestive system healthy
- Adequate exercise

If your cells don't have enough calcium, they will take the calcium from your bones, even at night. Sleeping is repair and recovery time.

COENZYME Q 10

The History of CoQ10

First discovered in 1857, CoQ10 has been met with lots of controversy due to the misunderstanding of this vital nutrient. Basically, CoQ10 is not a vitamin but a co-enzyme that greatly helps the other enzymes do their job in the body. An enzyme is a protein that while remaining unchanged itself, assists with chemical changes in other substances. It has been the subject of many impressive studies in Japan and Europe, where it is routinely used in the treatment of heart disease, especially congestive heart failure. But CoQ10 was almost completely ignored by the American medical community until now.

Coenzyme Q10 has been described as a "life-giving sparkplug" and is important in turning oxygen into pure energy. It is found in every cell in the body, except red blood cells. The unique antioxidant properties of CoQ10 are even more powerful than vitamin E and are astoundingly helpful in treating and preventing all kinds of cardiovascular problems, from arrhythmias to heart attacks, and even congestive heart failure. CoQ10 protects the heart from failure by keeping its energy levels high. But this nutraceutical doesn't just keep the heart pumping. Through its amazing energizing ability, CoQ10 can help treat illnesses as different as diabetes, chronic lung disease, and gum disease. One study even shows that the co-enzyme can reduce tumors associated with breast cancer. For those of us who are in good health, CoQ10 can improve fitness by increasing our exercise endurance.

Although our bodies can make CoQ10 in some situations, the body's capacity to produce CoQ10 isn't sufficient to meet its needs. CoQ10 levels reach their peak in the human body by the age twenty and fall slowly thereafter. In the US, 60% of the population in their fifties and sixties has CoQ10 deficiencies. In addition, certain medications, such as cholesterol-lowering drugs or statins, inhibit the body's production of CoenzymeQ10. Supplements can help, but since most supplemental CoQ10 is poorly absorbed by the body, a supplement must be highly bioavalable to be effective.

Benefits of CoQ10:
- Promotes heart health
- Prevents the oxidation of LDL cholesterol
- Provides energy at the cellular level
- Helps keep blood flowing freely through the arteries
- Helps in the treatment of breast cancer support during chemotherapy
- Treatment for Parkinson's
- Helps obesity
- Increases exercise tolerance

What the supplement must contain for best results:
- Uses all natural ingredients
- Must contain at least 30 mg. of Coenzyme Q10, 5 mg. of mixed tocopherols, and 640 mcg of Resveratrol in every capsule
- Needs clinical studies and patents for absorbability

VITAMIN D

Vitamin D was once very much overlooked but today is taking center stage on the prevention of health problems. It is important for good overall health and strong and healthy bones. It is also important for making sure your muscles, heart, lungs and brain work well and overall your body can resists/fight infection.

Here are D facts:

1. Our bodies make vitamin D from sunlight from a metabolite of cholesterol. This is different from other vitamins which must be acquired from food.

2. Vitamin D from sunlight and supplements has to be changed chemically in our body a number of times before it can be used. Then when it is ready, your body uses it to communicate with the blood, bones, gut and immune system to keep your body in balance.

3. For strong bones, calcium and phosphorus are essential for developing the structure and strength but need vitamin D to absorb these minerals. Even if you eat lots of calcium rich foods without adequate levels of vitamin D it will not be absorbed properly.

Vitamin D is essential for:

- A strong immune system – to fight infection.
- Muscle function.
- Cardiovascular function, for a healthy heart and circulation.
- Respiratory system – for healthy lungs and airways.
- Brain development.
- Anticancer effects - especially colon, breast, lung, and prostate cancer.
- Increasing the effectiveness of cancer treatment.
- Reducing incidence of asthma, type II diabetes, depression, Alzheimer's, autoimmune diseases like MS, Crohn's, Lupus, and Type I Diabetes.
- Lowering blood pressure (when combined with calcium and magnesium).
- Lowering the risk of developing Type I Diabetes in children.
- Helps cells all over your body to communicate.

There are more health benefits of getting enough vitamin D appearing in the literature every day.

How to get enough:

Sun

The most natural way is sun exposure – without sunscreen. Without needing to get a tan or burn just a few minutes daily can improve your vitamin D levels.

The amount of vitamin D you get from exposing your bare skin to the sun depends on:

- The time of day – your skin produces more vitamin D if you expose it during the middle of the day.
- Where you live – the closer to the equator you live, the easier it is for you to produce vitamin D from sunlight all year round.
- The color of your skin – pale skins make vitamin D more quickly than darker skins.
- The amount of skin you expose – the more skin your expose the more vitamin D your body will produce.

*From: www.vitamindcouncil.org

Supplementation

The other way is through supplementation. This is good even if you are getting adequate sun exposure. Vitamin D3 is the best kind to take and it comes in forms such as tablets and capsules. It does not matter what time of day you take it.

All calcium supplements should have D. Multivitamins should have D. Children's vitamins should have D. Look for natural food supplements that have raised the vitamin D level to meet the latest studies.

Most foods only contain small amounts of vitamin D so supplementing and sun exposure are the best resources.

Recommended and Upper Levels (UL) of daily intakes from various organizations:

	Vitamin D Council	Endocrine Society	Food and Nutrition Board
Infants	1,000 IU/day 2,000 UL	400-1,000 IU/day 2,000 UL	400 IU/day 1,500 UL
Children	1,000 IU/day per 25lbs of body weight 2,000 UL per 25 lbs. body wt.	600-1,000 IU/day 4,000 UL	600 IU/day 3,000 UL
Adults	5,000 IU/day 10,000 UL	1,500-2,000 IU/day 10,000 UL	600 IU/day, 800 IU/day for seniors 4,000 UL

Food
- Raw Milk
- Salmon
- Mackerel
- Tuna
- Sardines
- Egg yolks
- Beef liver

Get Your Score

Vitamin D is the essential of the essentials! It is what makes things happen in your body. Without it your immune system is like an army without weapons. Take time this month to make an appointment with your doctor to get your Vitamin D[25(OH)D] level checked. Then recheck every 3-6 months until you have reached the level of 100. Only by having your blood levels tested will you know if you are getting enough of this vital nutrient.

Vitamin D 25(OH)D range guidelines from various organizations:

	Vitamin D Council	Endocrine Society	Food and Nutrition Board	Testing Laboratories
Deficient	0-30 ng/ml	0-20 ng/ml	0-11 ng/ml	0-31 ng/ml
Insufficient	31-39 ng/ml	21-29 ng/ml	12-20 ng/ml	
Sufficient	40-80 ng/ml	30-100 ng/ml	>20 ng/ml	32-100 ng/ml
Toxic	>150 ng/ml			

VITAMIN E

If you had to choose two warriors to fight for your defense against free radical damage, your best choices would be Vitamins E and C. These two defenders pack a very powerful punch against the enemies while wearing the large "A" on their battle gear, which stands for antioxidant. They fight so that you don't have to even think about the invaders trying to take up refuge in your body.

What we call vitamin E is actually a family of compounds called tocopherols (which means to bring forth offspring) and tocotrienols.

What is Vitamin E, and what does it do?

Vitamin E:

- Is fat-soluble. It acts like an antioxidant and prevents pollution and toxins from entering the body.
- Helps with anti-aging—fewer wrinkles.
- Helps the body absorb other essential nutrients like Vitamin K and C.
- Regulates retinol—vitamin A—essential for skin and vision.
- Provides essential functions in cellular respiration of muscles.
- Aids in production of biological energy.
- Supports heart, prostate, lung, colon, and immune health.

Nature's Protector

Vitamin E is one of God's best known antioxidants. The presence of vitamin E helps protect other nutrients, such as vitamin A and the B vitamins, against oxidation. Although oxidation is a natural process, it must be controlled to avoid using up or destroying essential nutrients.

For example, you can compare the activity of vitamin E in your body's cells with the effect of using a sunscreen lotion on your skin. Just as a sunscreen helps control the tanning process, vitamin E helps control the harmful oxidation that occurs in cell membranes.

Vitamin E Helps Maintain Healthy Cell Membranes

Vitamin E may be an integral part of the cell membrane itself, lending it structural strength and stability. Many disease processes are associated with altered or abnormal cell membrane structure; therefore, maintaining healthful function in these membranes can be considered one of the most important aspects of health. Vitamin E can also "mop up" free radicals after they have been formed.

Vitamin E and Aging

Vitamin E may help slow the aging process of body cells by preventing the development of free radicals, which also occur as a result of chemical pollutants and radiation to which we are exposed daily. Aging is believed to be due to the gradual accumulation of the destructive results of free radicals in the system. Enzymes can't function, cell's energy sources become crippled, and cells can't fight back and they begin to die—and there aren't enough replacements. Thus the aging process advances.

It is well-established that the membrane of the red blood cell is weakened in a vitamin E deficiency, resulting in the rupture of the cell membrane. Vitamin E and selenium together are believed to help strengthen the cell and prevent its rupture.

Vitamin E and Air Pollution

In the respiratory system, E protects the lungs and bronchial tubes from air pollution. In an atmosphere created to simulate air pollution in the city, lung tissue in animals was monitored. With the normal amount of E found in the American diet, lung damage was found to severe levels. When the E was increased to double the normal amount, lung damage was almost non-existent.

Vitamin E—The Heart and Muscle Builder

- Muscles and their nerves (especially cardiac and skeletal muscles) can function with less oxygen, thereby increasing their endurance and stamina.
- Decreases the oxygen requirement of a muscle (the heart is a muscle) by at least 43%, enabling the body to do the same job on less oxygen.
- Causes dilation of blood vessels, permitting a fuller flow of blood to the heart.
- Highly effective anti-thrombin in the bloodstream, inhibiting coagulation of blood by preventing clots from forming.
- Increases energy, speed, and endurance, and athletes the world over are now routinely being given vitamin E to improve their performance.

Selenium and Synergy; Vitamin E Sister Act

Selenium, an essential trace mineral, works "synergistically" with vitamin E for greater nutritional benefit. The effect of both being available to the body at the same time is greater than if they were separate. Simple but true, synergy means 1+1=3.

In a recent study, selenium supplementation (200mcg/day) was found to decrease the incidence of prostate cancer by more than 60%.

In a large intervention trial for skin cancer, the surprise finding was those people who took supplemental selenium had a 37% decrease in prostate, colorectal, and lung cancer as well as a 50% reduction in cancer deaths.

In a 1983 multi-institutional study, those patients treated with selenium had only about one-third as many prostate tumors as the patients receiving the placebo. In addition, there were no toxic effects of selenium supplementation.

What to Look for in a Vitamin E/ Selenium Supplement:

- Needs to include: alpha, beta, gamma, and delta tocopherols plus tocotrienols, selenium, and grape seed extract. Anything less is like leaving out part of the recipe.
- Package should state "d-alpha tocopherol." The form d-alpha tocopherol is the most biologically effective of all the natural tocopherols. The "d" means the element is from natural, not chemical, sources.
- Should *not* state "dl-tocopherol." This is a petrochemical synthetic form and harmful

to your health.
- Comes primarily from soybeans and wheat germ oil.
- Selenium is necessary for Vitamin E absorption.

Foods rich in Vitamin E:
- Wheat Germ
- Nuts and Seeds
- Spinach and other greens
- Organic Corn
- Asparagus

EFA—ESSENTIAL FATTY ACIDS

Beautiful hair, soft skin, soft un-calloused feet, eyes that are not dry, and nails that shine – all this is result of healthy fats in the diet. There was a day when experts said we were fat because we ate fat but yet today no one would dare make such a claim. The body loves healthy fats. The essential fatty acids necessary for health, cannot be made by the body, and must be supplied through the diet.

The body requires healthy sources of fat for:

- Basic structure of hormones.
- Cushioning body organs and keeping us warm.
- A concentrated source of energy.
- Healthy brain, nerve, and heart tissues.
- Healthy skin, nails, hair, and bones.
- All organ and glandular functions.
- Cellular communication.
- Cell growth, division, and repair.
- Absorption and transportation of fat-soluble vitamins.
- Building blocks of cell membranes.
- Production of prostaglandins—hormone-like substances that act as chemical messengers and regulators of various body processes.

Two basic categories of essential fatty acids:
1. *Omega-3**—Flax seeds, hemp oil, pumpkin seeds, walnut oils, deepwater fish, dark leafy vegetables, organic canola and organic soy

*Note—very high amounts of Omega-3 are found in commercial grade oils and virtually all processed food, *but* these have been converted into "bad" trans-fats through their high heat processing methods.

2. *Omega-6*—Borage oil, evening primrose oil, soy, hemp, black currant oil, nuts, seeds, grape seed, sesame, seeds, peanuts, sunflower seeds, safflower, legumes

Omega-6 and Omega-3 must be consumed in the correct balance to properly manage the three types of prostaglandins and to maintain optimal health. Omega 6 is a powerful protector when consumed in the correct proportions and combined with omega 3. When we consume too much omega 6 our blood tends to get sticky (viscosity) and clots.

Correcting the balance of EFA's:
- Eliminate hydrogenated oils.
- Eliminate poor quality Omega-6 sources, roasted or cooked seeds and nuts.
- Increase good quality Omega-6 sources.
- Increase intake of Omega-3 (flax seed, GLA, fish oils).
- Must have proper amounts of zinc, vitamin B, vitamin C and magnesium for the body to correctly assimilate EFA.
- See the reading on Flax Seed and GLA.

EPA—Eicosapetaenoic Acid—Essential Fatty Acid

The Benefits:
- Reduces triglycerides
- Reduces cholesterol
- Lowers blood pressure, if needed
- Reduces platelet adhesiveness and blood viscosity
- Lowers risk of cardiovascular disease (disease of the heart and blood vessels)
- Increases brain function
- Improves blood sugar metabolism
- Improves joint health
- Improves pregnancy health and child development
- Improves ADHD, autism, developmental coordination disorder, learning disabilities and poor cognitive abilities

EPA—What Is It?
EPA, eicosapetaenoic acid, is an essential fatty acid found in cold water "blue-scale" fish. EPA and its partner, DHA, are known as omega-3 fatty acids. They are not produced by the body and can only be acquired through diet or supplementation. Most fats consumed in the Western diet are omega-6 fatty acids. While omega-6 fatty acids contribute to the formation

of plaque in the arteries, which leads to the constriction of arterial walls, omega-3 fatty acids have been shown to actually reduce the risk of plaque formation and the subsequent problems associated with it.

The History

For years, scientist have studied heart disease and tried to find the clue to the mystery of cholesterol and fats. The controversy pits animals fats (mostly saturated) against vegetable fats (usually unsaturated), and animal fats continue to play the role of the villain. Yet, some cultures consume diets rich in animal fats and remain virtually free of heart disease. The Eskimos and the coastal Japanese are two examples of people who have traditionally eaten large quantities of animal fats and maintain an extremely low incidence of cardiovascular disease.

What is the missing link? High consumption of cold saltwater fish known as "blue-scale" fish, such as salmon, mackerel, sardines, and anchovies.

Interestingly, when Westerners are given diets high in these fish, blood changes occur that resemble the protective blood of the Eskimo. Unfortunately, to consume enough of these fish to get the needed fatty acids from them would require large quantities on a daily basis. After more research, the fatty acids found in these fish were isolated and extracted and are now available in supplement form. The two primary fatty acids, EPA and DHA, seem to work together to set up a series of beneficial conditions within the body that reduce the risk of cardiovascular disease.

> After years of research, we now know that omega-3 fatty acids are absolutely required by the body. They're not optional nutrients. Yet most of the population is deficient in them. The consumption of cholesterol and fat is way up at a time when omega-3 consumption is way down. We obviously need these fatty acids more than ever. They're the last major nutrient family to be recognized. In more ways than one, they're our nutritional missing link.
>
> ~Donald O. Rudin, M. D.[43]

What to Look for in Fish Oil Supplements

Unfortunately, not all fish oil products are safe and effective, as many factors can negatively affect the formula. This makes the processing technology utilized to purify the formula absolutely critical. Be sure to check with the company manufacturing the product to see if they guarantee that there are no contaminants or heavy metals in the supplement. With the high incidence of contamination off the shores of most continents, the fish is a better quality in the deeper oceans, away from shore. The company you purchase a supplement from should be able to tell you their source and if they are using smaller, less-contaminated fish for their supplements.

When looking for a supplement, check to see that they are using a molecular distillation process to remove all contaminants and to retain the quality of seven naturally-occurring essential fatty acids: EPA, DHA, ALA, docosapantaenoic, stearidonic, eicosatetraenoic, and henelcosapentaenoic.

Similar but *not* Equal: Fish Oil vs. Flaxseed

Since flaxseed oil contains concentrated amounts of omega-3 fatty acids, some patients are confusing the benefits of flaxseed oil with fish oil. Although they are similar in structure, the omega-3s in flaxseed, alpha-linolenic acid (ALA), is a precursor or "parent" to the omega-3s that are found directly in fish oil, EPA and DHA. In your body, ALA converts poorly into EPA and into DHA. Typically, this means between seven to eleven grams of flaxseed is needed to produce the same benefits as one gram of fish oil. Of course, eating foods high in ALA is much better than not receiving any omega-3 fatty acids at all.

Omega-3 Fatty Acids
- Beneficial for rheumatoid arthritis
- Good for all forms of arthritis
- Help control viral infections
- Reduce cholesterol and triglycerides
- Lower the risk of stroke or heart attack
- Reduce the risk of arteriosclerosis
- Improve psoriasis
- Improve immune response
- Lower harmful effects of prostaglandins, aiding in preventing breast cancer
- Reduce severity of migraine headaches
- Improve brain function
- Improve function of the glandular system

FLAVONOIDS

When you think of flavonoids, think in colors. While our carotenoids are rich in orange, yellow, and red-orange foods, our flavonoids are rich in blue, purple, or red colors. This is not exclusive but a good rule to follow with your diet—make it colorful.

More than 4,000 chemically unique flavonoids are known. Foods rich in these phytochemicals include:

Beets	Blackberries
Blueberries	Cherries
Purple and red grapes	Purple cabbage

Spices   Bilberries
Green Tea

Benefits of flavonoids:

Cancer protective   Connective tissue regeneration
Anti-inflammatory   Promote blood flow
Reduce cholesterol   Antioxidants
Promote collagen formation

The best results for bolstering the immune system occur when a complex mixture and variety of phytonutrients are consumed either in the diet or in the form of nutritional supplements.

Flavonoids directly support the immune system and can act as antibiotics. They have anti-inflammatory and anti-cancer action. Studies have demonstrated that flavonoids actually inhibit the growth of blood vessels in tumors. They are beneficial in maintaining a healthy heart by helping to prevent blood clots and generally improve vascular health. This causes a reduction in the risk of not only heart disease but also strokes. Flavonoids help prevent certain forms of cancer by inducing death in malignant cells, help prevent osteoporosis, and even decrease the symptoms of allergies.

Flavonoids are water soluble. A flavonoid supplement needs to have all six flavonoid classes:

- Anthocyanadins   - Proanthocynadins
- Polyphenols   - Flavanones
- Flavones   - Flavonols

Finally, remember that the carotenoids and the flavonoids are complementary.

GARLIC

Medical History

Garlic's medical history is fascinating. The early actions ascribed to garlic are the very same ones we find mentioned in modern medical literature.

From Hippocrates (370 B.C.) to the Roman Era, to the doctors in England in 1812, the findings were the same. Garlic:

- Promotes urination (diuretic).
- Reestablishes microflora.
- Reduces inflammation.
- Aids in the stomach (digestive aid).
- Clears the lungs, bronchial tubes, and throat (an expectorant).

- Clears the blood (lowers cholesterol).
- Helps with pus (antibiotic).
- Could reduce a fever, produce sweating, and aid in regulating menstruation.

Garlic is still used for these purposes today. What drug do we know of with a 2,000 year history of continual success? Throughout the centuries of history, the studies of garlic have remained consistent and continue to bring health benefits.

Just what is garlic?

What does it contain to have all of these wonderful properties? How does garlic suddenly develop its characteristic odor and taste? Take a clove of garlic, peel it, and you get no odor. Lick it, and there is no taste. Boil without cutting and you get a vegetable taste. The strong odor and taste appear only after it has been crushed or cut.

Here is the secret: Two substances in the bulb are kept away from each other in the normal undisturbed bulb. They are alliin and alliinase. Alliinase is an enzyme that is released when the bulb is cut or crushed. It acts on alliin to form a thin compound called allicin. This is the major active compound of garlic. It has the strong smell and taste we commonly describe as "garlicky."

Allicin is an unstable compound and soon breaks down into two other compounds that still have health benefits. Then in a matter of hours or days, it begins to change into compounds called sulfides. They have lessened health benefits. With more time, you finally end up with some seventy polysulfides, which have a smell but no health benefits.

Is there much research?

Garlic is very well studied. On the medical computer bank, you can find an astounding 700 articles published in the last twenty years, confirming the benefits of garlic.

Infections in General

Garlic has a strong reputation for combating bacterial infections, especially throat, ear, chest, mouth, diarrhea, bronchitis, and sinus problems. Garlic can slow or kill more than sixty fungi and twenty types of bacteria. Another big plus for garlic is that, as far as we know, bacterial resistance does not develop.

Respiratory Problems

Moscow had a massive influenza epidemic in 1965. The power of garlic in respiratory problems was so well accepted by the medical community that they spent a lot of rubles for an emergency airlift of 500 metric tons. The influenza epidemic was stopped cold.

In Eastern Europe, professionals in respiratory problems often use garlic where antibiotics would be prescribed in the West. When you do get colds, bronchitis, sinusitis, and sore throats, get rest, drink a lot of water, and take vitamin C; but by all means, add garlic. Garlic encourages mucous secretions and helps open clogged and swollen mucous membranes. It works so well that the Ministry of Health in the United Kingdom issued a license for garlic. It allows manufacturers of garlic products to claim it is traditionally used for the treatment of all of the inflammatory respiratory problems I just mentioned.

Candida Invasions

Candida infections seem to be on the rise in our culture for one reason or another. Studies from all over the world have shown garlic to be very effective. Garlic is now the number one treatment for Candida. If you have a serious or resistant case, obviously you are going to need pharmaceutical support. But once free of Candida, it would be foolish to ever stop taking garlic.

The Anti-infective Ingredient

Without a doubt, it is the allicin. Remember that allicin begins to break down as soon as the bulb is damaged. Be sure that whatever garlic product you take contains all of the potential allicin of the fresh bulb to get the full garlic power.

Circulatory Diseases

As most of us know, heart and circulatory diseases are the number one killers of Americans. Some of the contributing factors are: high cholesterol, edema, high blood pressure, and blood that clots too quickly. The good news is that garlic works to improve all of these listed problems. In addition, in Germany, garlic is a licensed medicine for atherosclerosis.

In a survey of the best studies, you will find that you can expect an amazing drop in cholesterol of anywhere from 10 to 20%. Over 66% of Americans have a cholesterol count somewhat above the range for optimal health. They are often the ones "lost through the cracks." It's not enough for the doctor to prescribe a drug, but it is high enough for concern. A safe, mild, totally natural product, such as a quality garlic supplement, could radically alter this situation.

The Fast Clot

Americans have a blood clotting time that is too fast for our 21st century circulatory epidemic. As of 1992, the speed of the blood clot is listed as a risk factor with smoking, high cholesterol, and high blood pressure. You see, in some 90% of heart attacks, a blood clot is responsible. Garlic's action on the prostaglandins that control parts of blood clotting helps the body not to form clots inside blood vessels. The effect is similar to aspirin, which many doctors recommend to slow the blood clot. But there is one exception: garlic does not have the side effects of aspirin.

High Blood Pressure

Reducing high blood pressure is another action of garlic. In reviewing thirteen high blood pressure studies, I found that the average drop in diastolic blood pressure consistently ranges from 5–10%.

Cancer and Garlic

Garlic is a powerful antioxidant, and it has some anti-cancer properties. It contains significant amounts of selenium and germanium, plus several amino acids that all protect us from free radicals. It is thought that some of the many sulfur compounds also give protection.

The National Cancer Institute did very thorough studies in China concerning stomach cancer. The Shandong province has a very high rate of stomach cancer. NCI found that those Chinese who ate garlic on a regular basis were only 40% as likely to develop cancer as those who did not eat garlic.

Heavy metal

Heavy metal contamination, such as lead and mercury seems to be a rising problem in our society. The many sulfur compounds in garlic can trap these metals and take them to elimination.

Mercury is a very toxic metal. In one animal study, mercury was given to rats. Animals consuming garlic eliminated it two to three times faster than those not consuming garlic. For those concerned about mercury fillings, taking garlic should give some peace of mind.

More benefits

There are numerous reports indicating that garlic can help diabetes. It seems to work better in type 2 or adult onset diabetes.

Other actions of garlic that are mentioned from time to time in the literature are: stimulating the immune system, easing menstrual cramps, reducing flatulence, aiding muscle cramps, helping cold hands and feet, and having a positive effect on aging.

Garlic Supplements

There are numerous garlic supplements on the market today. Keep in mind that the undisturbed garlic bulb has potential powerful health-promoting components. As soon as it is disturbed, the breakdown process begins.

Obviously, raw, fresh garlic is the easiest and cheapest way to consume this product. Unfortunately, it may not be the best way to obtain garlic's benefits. Some people do not like the strong taste, especially with their breakfast cereal. For others, fresh garlic can cause an uncomfortable but temporary sensation of nausea. For still other people, the odor of garlic on the breath can be quite disturbing, leading possibly to the loss of friends, relatives, and others dear to you. A few people are sensitive to raw garlic and can develop a skin rash from handling the cloves. To assure consistent potency and a measured delivery of beneficial materials, garlic should be consumed in a food supplement form. This can give you the assurance that you are getting all the active compounds you need to promote and protect your health.

There are six basic ways to prepare a garlic supplement:

- *Garlic oil capsules, crushed garlic,* and *conventional high heat:* The problem with these three is that much of the allicin is lost, thereby reducing the effectiveness.
- *Freeze–dried powder:* Cold and intense heat is used for a shorter time than with the conventional high-heat method. The allicin content is reduced by less than the conventional method. The problem is that this is an expensive product, and you can get a better supplement at a lesser price.
- *Temperature-controlled or cool-dried:* This is a unique process. The whole garlic bulb is exposed to near-room-temperature air for about thirty minutes. This process results in a dry powder with all the original allicin. Remember, this is the pre-allicin material of the fresh garlic. The allicin is not converted to allicin until the product is dissolved or digested. Since the allicin is created during digestion, and most digestion takes place past the stomach, there is little after-odor. These tablets are odor controlled. This product has several advantages over the others we have mentioned. It is mild to the stomach. The potency very closely resembles the raw, fresh garlic. The final product contains almost 100% of the potential allicin, vitamins, minerals, and other natural ingredients.
- *Aged odorless extracts:* These were quite popular because of the cost and the fact that they were odor-free. They are made by chopping garlic and aging it in alcohol for long periods of time before extracting the contents. The powders produced by this process contain additives or must be freeze-dried, and this inhibits the level of active ingredients in the material. Many of these products do not contain the main garlic ingredient, allicin. Also, as the product undergoes disintegration, it does not produce some of the active sulfur compounds. This raises some real questions about the medical activity.

Summary of supplements: Look for a pure, natural, and pesticide-free product. It should be odor-controlled, and the best process is the cool-dried or temperature-controlled process. The label should state how much garlic is in each capsule or tablet. It should tell you how many capsules equal one clove so you can easily choose your dose.[44, 45]

GLA

GLA, Gamma Linoleic Acid, is one of two essential fatty acids—Omega-3 and Omega-6—fats that are necessary for maintaining normal functioning and growth of cells, nerves, muscles, and organs. Omega-6 is also involved in the communication that leads to the production of prostaglandins in the body. Prostaglandins are a potent, hormone-like substance that helps regulate numerous bodily processes. The body uses prostaglandins to control inflammation, dilate blood vessels, and regulate immune function.

Many researchers believe that Omega-3 is deficient in many people but that Omega-6 is very prevalent in our diets due to the common vegetable oils that contain this fat. Besides evening primrose oil, other sources of GLAs include borage oil and black currant seed oil. Omega-6 can also be found in meats, milk, and eggs.

Studies show we are suffering from many symptoms (as listed below) because our bodies are unable to convert the Omega-6 to GLA. This poor conversion may be due to diet, alcohol, and diabetes.

GLA helps alleviate the following:

- ADHD
- Breast Tenderness
- Diabetes
- Eczema
- High blood cholesterol
- Immune dysfunction
- Issues with clotting of blood
- MS
- Pain
- PMS*** Yes this really works
- Problems with blood pressure
- Rheumatoid arthritis
- Alcoholism
- Chronic Fatigue
- Dry eyes
- Fertility issues
- High edema in pregnancy
- Inflammation
- Issues with hair loss
- Osteoporosis
- Periodontitis
- Poor libido
- Psoriasis

In addition, GLA provides good prostate support, improves sexual hormonal response and skin and nail health, increases metabolic rate, and protects cells from damaging trans-fats.

Best to look for:

Borage oil—highest potency and best bioavailability, can be mixed with Sunflower oil in a capsule. Borage seed oil has 2.5 times as much GLA as Evening Primrose Oil. The product needs to be cold pressed to retain natural character. The bottle may not say this, so you may have to ask the company to determine if they are acquiring this oil through the cold pressed method.

Personal note:

Many people have seen great results in inflammation being reduced, eczema going away, and for women, the return of sexual desire for their husbands. This supplement does not work overnight, but as you continue to take it, you may notice an improvement. If you are taking it for libido problems, then you will probably need to continue on this supplement to get the desired results. One person told me her husband says that GLA stands for "got lucky again."

IRON

Every cell in the body contains and requires iron. This mineral is needed for all body functions which is why it is guarded by the body and when depleted causes symptoms.

Symptoms of Iron deficiency:
- Anorexia
- Brittle nails
- Compromised immune system
- Constipation
- Decreased attention span in children/decreased play
- Difficult breathing
- Fatigue
- Headaches
- Impaired concentration
- Lethargy
- Lower IQs in children
- Pale looking skin
- Tendencies of hyperactivity in children
- Tiredness

Iron deficiency is usually caused by insufficient intake in our diets. It can also be caused by intestinal bleeding caused by medications, poor digestion, ulcers, heavy perspiring, antacids, and heavy drinking of coffee and/or caffeine.

Who Needs Iron?
- Boys and girls, especially infants 2–24 months
- Pre-menopausal women
- Those over 55 years old
- Some men

- Some low-income people
- Athletes and other people who engage in vigorous physical activities
- Anyone who has recently had surgery
- Anyone under stress for long periods of time
- ** Microwaved foods have been proven to lower white blood cells, which then weakens the immune system and can then lead to anemia.

Benefits of Iron
- Prevents anemia
- Stimulates bone-marrow production of red blood cells
- Forms part of several enzymes and protein in the body

What to Look for in a Supplement*
If you are unable to get enough iron in your diet, then a supplement may be necessary. There are certain guidelines to look for when choosing a supplement.

- Look for ferrous fumarate. This is less toxic, less irritating, better absorbed, and more stable than the other salts of iron.
- Vitamin C increases the absorption of iron by 30%. It is best if this is combined with the iron in one tablet.
- Iron is best absorbed 45 minutes away from a dairy food.

*Don't take iron in a supplement if you have hepatitis or excess iron in your body.

LECITHIN

Benefits of Lecithin
- Heart—cholesterol, triglycerides, circulation
- Brain—functioning and learning—ADD/ADHD, hyperactivity, dementia
- Weight loss—"fat gobbler," breaking down fats, redistributing body fats
- Joints—lubricates joints and intestinal lining
- Liver—softens hardened liver tissue, improves bile flow

Note: Lecithin is used as a thickener in foods. When reading labels on your food, make sure it is a soy lecithin added; otherwise, lecithin could be a petroleum-based ingredient.

Foods containing Lecithin
All animal and plant products contain lecithin, including:

- Cabbage
- Eggs
- Garbanzo beans
- Green beans
- Seeds/nuts
- Soy lecithin
- Wheat germ

- Cauliflower
- Fish
- Grains
- Lentils
- Soy beans
- Split peas

Nature's Gatekeeper

Lecithin, a phospholipid, is needed in every cell in the body. It is found in all cell membranes and body tissues, including the brain, liver, and heart. Lecithin plays a vital role in nutrient transportation in and out of the cells and therefore may be called the "gatekeeper" of the cell. If phospholipids are not present in sufficient amounts to maintain the cell membrane structure, the membrane loses its ability to protect and nourish the cell.

Nature's Emulsifier

Lecithin, like EPA, is an essential fatty acid. It cannot be manufactured by the body and is necessary to health. Lecithin has earned the nickname "nature's emulsifier" because of its ability to hold fat molecules in a solution.

Oil and water don't mix, but lecithin's molecular structure allows it to unite with both, solving the problem of absorbing fats and the fat-soluble vitamins into the water-based body.

A Key to Absorption of Vitamins

Lecithin, along with other substances, is used by the liver to make yellowish-orange fluid called bile. Bile is concentrated and stored in a sac called the gallbladder. During digestion, the bile from the gallbladder and liver is pumped into the small intestines, where it emulsifies fat and fat-soluble nutrients, like essential fatty acids and vitamins A, D, and E. This emulsion facilitates the absorption of these nutrients into the body.

An Aid in Dieting

Because so many nutrients fall under the category of "fat," there is confusion about which are needed and which are to be avoided. It is important not to make the mistake of avoiding all fat.

Essential fatty acids are just that, essential. Lecithin acts as a solvent for cholesterol and other fats and, as such, draws deposits of fat into the bloodstream, where the extra fat is chemically burned. Because of this, some doctors believe it is one of the most important nutrients to be included in a fat-reducing diet. Even distribution of the body weight may also be aided by lecithin.

Looking for Choline and Inositol

Choline, found in lecithin, is needed for the proper transmission of nerve impulses from the brain through the central nervous system, as well as for gallbladder function and liver health. A deficiency of this substance can cause actual brain disorders. A number of studies have shown that in some cases learning disabilities, nervous afflictions, and even some early senility yielded to doses of lecithin.

Choline is important to the nerves, for it's a component of the myelin sheath that surrounds and insulates nerve fibers. Choline apparently exerts a protective action in cirrhosis of the liver among alcoholics and helps maintain healthy kidneys jeopardized by heavy drinking.

Inositol, also found in lecithin, helps choline perform its vital functions and also promotes healthy hair, helps prevent eczema, has a calming effect, helps to reduce cholesterol levels, and aids in redistribution of body fat.

Sources of Lecithin

Lecithin can be found in the health food store as a liquid, powder, or a supplement. The liquid can be used to coat your baking pans to help them not stick. The liquid and powder can be added to any recipe for added health benefits. The supplement can be added to your diet and is usually found in a gel form.

MAGNESIUM

Important for:
- Altitude sickness
- Chemical toxicity
- Converting vitamin D to its active form
- Fibromyalgia
- Headache
- High blood pressure
- Kidney function
- Over 300 enzyme reactions
- Pregnancy – reduces rate of eclampsia
- Premenstrual syndrome
- Preventing/ treating heart disease and strokes/ mitral valve prolapse
- Prevents kidney stones formation
- Treating and preventing osteoporosis
- Treating asthma
- Type 1 Diabetics

Deficiency causes
- Taking diuretics such as Lasix, aspirin therapy
- Diabetes
- Poor kidney function
- Pancreatitis
- Laxative use
- Cardiac bypass surgery
- Digestive disorders
- Caffeine use
- Diarrhea
- Major burns,
- High sodium diets

Symptoms of deficiency
- Fatigue
- Muscle weakness
- Increases complications in diabetes, heart disease, osteoporosis, preeclampsia, asthma, renal stones

Foods High in Magnesium
- Almonds
- Barley
- Beets
- Brussels sprouts
- Brown rice
- Cauliflower
- Collard greens
- Cornmeal
- Lentils
- Milk
- Millet
- Oats
- Peanut butter
- Peas
- Sesame seeds
- Sweet potato
- Tomato
- White beans
- Asparagus
- Beet greens
- Black-eyed peas
- Broccoli
- Carrot or onion
- Cashews
- Corn
- Green pepper
- Lima beans
- Milk
- Mushrooms
- Peanut butter
- Peanuts
- Red beans
- Spinach
- Swiss chard
- Wheat bran/germ

PROBIOTICS

Bring in the "good" guys and destroy the "bad." A battle is raging within you, whether you know it or not, so the question is: do you need to get armed and ready or sit back and watch? That is the question everyone should be asking. But first, let's define what probiotics are and why we need them.

Did you know that probiotics can:

- Be our first line of defense for immune system health?
- Help fight Candida?
- Protect your entire digestive tract?
- Break down fecal material and help to prevent colon cancer and polyps?

Probiotics are Intestinal Microflora. Microflora is the term used to describe the organisms (bacteria) that live in the intestinal tract. These bacteria are responsible for numerous essential bodily functions. The colon has about two to three pounds of bacterial organisms calling it home. Of those three pounds of bacteria, there needs to be a ratio of 80% good guys and no more than 20% of the bad guys. When this is out of balance and the bad guys are winning, you may have any of the following symptoms:

- Any immune issues
- Athlete's foot
- Candida
- Colitis
- Constipation/diarrhea
- Cravings
- Crohn's
- Digestive issues
- Food poisoning
- IBS/ IBD
- Infections – ear, abscess, wounds, fungal, tonsillitis
- Skin issues
- Thrush
- Typical sore throat
- Unexplained weight loss
- Yeast infections

Good microflora are destroyed by:

- Physical and emotional stress.
- Unhealthy lifestyle choices—lack of physical activity, smoking, low-fiber diets, too much alcohol, negative attitudes.
- Food and water contaminants—chemical preservatives in our water (including fluoride and chlorine) and food, processed foods, and hormones in food.
- Antibiotics and medications—aspirin, steroids, laxatives
- Estrogen—birth control pills and prescription estrogen
- Travel
- Stress—emotional and physical

Overcome the Imbalance by:

- Eating a healthful diet with fermented foods such as yogurt, sauerkraut and kefir.
- Exercising consistently.
- Drinking ½ your body weight in ounces of purified water every day.
- Getting adequate rest.
- Trying to control stress.
- Taking a probiotic supplement.

What do good bacteria do for us?

Good bacteria:

- Produce important B vitamins, also known as anti-stress vitamins.
- Manufacture the enzyme lactase, which helps digest dairy products.
- Improve digestive efficiency and proper bowel function.
- Recycle toxins.
- Reduce cholesterol levels by contributing to cholesterol metabolism and utilization.
- Stimulate a powerful immune system.
- In order to claim their territory, can deactivate disease-causing bacteria—the Bad Guys.
- Can produce their own antibiotic-like substances, which can kill invading bacteria, viruses, and yeast.

The good guys as well as the bad guys continuously die off and are eliminated from the body. It is vital to continually replenish your supply of good bacteria to offset the bad bacteria that make their way into your system via food, air, water, etc.

Feed the Troops

Prebiotics feed the probiotics. Prebiotic fiber that would enhance the growth of the probiotics include fiber mainly from fruits and vegetables, asparagus, carrots, onions, garlic, green and black tea, honey and chicory root. Ideally everyone should aim for 4-12 cups of vegetables per day.

Who needs to take a supplement?

Considering the large amount of chemicals in our air, water, food, and cleaners, everyone needs to be taking a probiotic supplement. If not on a continuous basis, then you might want to consider it when issues arise with your immune system or when you are taking prescriptions, traveling, or having digestive issues.

What to Look for in a Supplement

There are many brands and types of probiotics on the market. Even in your favorite stores that you shop frequently and trust, you will find probiotics that are not worth the money spent on them. The label must say *"guaranteed live delivery through expiration date."* Many products will only say "live bacteria at time of manufacture." Look for a probiotic that comes in a triple encapsulated form and guarantees live human strain bacteria.

PROTEIN AS A SUPPLEMENT

Meat, eggs, and cheese are typically what comes to mind when people think protein. One of the biggest sellers of protein is not an animal product but powders sold in the health food stores, gyms and supplement suppliers. But why do people purchase protein as a supplement when it is so prevalent in our meals? As we all know America eats the most meat of any country but yet many Americans are malnourished or protein deficient. Because of this many sports enthusiasts, weight loss candidates and others are buying the powder expecting great results.

Listed here are the five types of protein supplements on the market for five different reasons[47]. Personally I do not start my day without the protein powder called 180 ™. 180 gives me a balanced supply of protein, fiber, and carbohydrates, along with a good supply of vitamins and minerals. It is a perfect start to a great day without any GMO or artificial ingredients.

The most important reason to add a high quality protein supplement is that every single cell in your body requires protein to build. This means we need to have it in our diet at every meal.

1. *A vegetable-based (soy or rice) supplement:* This is used primarily to add extra protein to your diet. A good organic soy protein drink is sweetened with fructose and glucose, both naturally occurring in fruits and vegetables. The essential amino

acids should be listed on the label. This is a high-quality protein and low fat health insurance.

2. *A complete meal replacement*: Most of the time this is a nonfat, dry milk-based product. It should contain a full complement of vitamins and minerals to make it a complete meal replacement.

3. *A weight loss supplement*: This is usually a protein mix of milk protein and soy protein isolate. It can be used as a meal replacement. Of all the protein supplements, it is most important for the one for weight loss to be in perfect balance for your body. It should be powerful enough to be mixed with plain water in case you are not around cold milk. The drink should also contain a minimum of 4 grams of fiber. This helps you feel full longer. One serving in plain water should give about 15 grams of protein, 3 grams of fat, and around 210 calories.

4. *For the serious Athlete*: A good supplement would be a milk protein-based (whey) product that is precisely designed and clinically tested to give faster energy return, increased muscle mass, and strength. This category would also include those doing hard physical labor, yard work, or garage cleanups; those recovering from surgery, injury, or illness; and those in physical therapy for neuron—muscular disorders. In all these activities, a good product can help you suffer less soreness and have better endurance, faster recovery, and more energy.

5. *A drink for those who work out regularly*: This should be a milk protein-based drink that is specifically designed for energy recovery and fuel for tired, hungry muscles. This drink should contain 12 grams of protein, 33 grams of carbohydrates, 0.5 grams of fat, and around 180 calories.

When purchasing a protein supplement, be sure there is published science to back up the claims of the product. A lot of statements on muscle building products are sales pitch and pure "hype." Look for a reputable company with a 100% guarantee.

What to Look for in a Good Supplement:
- It should contain no artificial sweeteners, flavors, preservatives, or colors. These do nothing for health.
- It should be a quality protein with a high level of biological availability. Under the FDA standard for assessing protein quality, the pattern of the nine essential amino acids in a protein is compared to the actual human requirements of these amino acids. Then an adjustment is applied based on how well the proteins digested. Organic soy protein has been given a score of one, the highest possible rating, and is equal to animal proteins such as those from free range eggs and organic milk.

- Low in fat
- 99% lactose free
- It should contain no hormones, antibiotics, or other dangerous chemicals.
- There should be minimal cholesterol.
- Preparation should be easy. It should mix in water, milk, or juice for convenience.
- Except for a muscle building product, the supplement should be low enough in calories to be useful in a weight reduction or weight maintenance program.
- There should be no superlative claims on the can or literature such as "lose weight while you sleep" or "massive muscles in 30 days" or other statements.

SAW PALMETTO

The Saw Palmetto berry extract is an herbal product that may be used for men's health. When looking for a supplement, look for a complex containing Beta-sitosterol, Pumpkin Seed Oil, and soybeans. A supplement should not contain Hexane. This is a toxic ingredient.

The purpose of Saw Palmetto is to maintain proper urinary flow, support the prostate gland, and to support male sexual health. It acts as a diuretic, urinary antiseptic, and appetite stimulant. It inhibits the production of dihydrotestosterone, a form of testosterone that contributes to enlargement of the prostate. It may also enhance sexual functioning and desire. It has been used clinically to treat benign prostate hyperplasia. It is an anti-inflammatory and potential immune stimulant. Consider these recent studies[48]

- Many European studies have shown that Saw Palmetto improves symptoms of benign prostate hyperplasia (BPH), an enlargement of the prostate that causes uncomfortable urinary symptoms as men get older. Symptoms include difficult urination, incomplete emptying of the bladder and a frequent urge to urinate.
- Recently, the first American clinical trial confirmed these results and showed that this plant also reduced swelling in enlarged prostate tissue.
- In a study of 305 patients with mild to moderate symptoms of BPH, supplementation with 160 milligrams of Saw Palmetto twice a day resulted in an 88% reduction of symptoms.
- An earlier double-blind study found the following results after just one month of treatment: 47% decrease in nightly bathroom visits, 50% increase in urinary flow, and 42% reduction in residual urine.
- Saw palmetto works by inhibiting the enzyme, 5-alpha reductase, which converts testosterone to its more active form, dihydrotestosterone (DHT) and it also blocks the binding of this hormone to receptor sites on the prostate.

- It also increases the breakdown and excretion of DHT and helps stop the pain and inflammation associated with BPH.

Note: It can take up to 4–8 weeks for maximum benefits.

PUMPKIN SEEDS

Pumpkin seeds actually contain more iron than liver by weight. Pumpkin seeds are an excellent source of essential fatty acids that promote good prostaglandin production. A popular treatment for prostate problems, pumpkin seeds are a popular herbal remedy that can be used as a mild laxative with additional diuretic action. The reason this topic is included here is that pumpkin seeds are typically included in many men's health supplements. When combined with saw palmetto, beta Sitosterol and organic soybeans this can be sold as a complete prostate supplement.

Key nutrients in pumpkin seeds:

- Calcium
- Fiber
- Magnesium
- Phosphorus
- Protein
- Sodium
- Zinc

- Copper
- Iron
- Manganese
- Potassium
- Selenium
- Vitamins A, B, C and E.

They are high in polyunsaturated and monounsaturated fatty acids and both essential and nonessential amino acids. The phytochemicals in them include phytosterols.

ZINC

Benefits of Zinc:
- Healthy immune functions
- Healing of wounds
- Anti-inflammatory
- Maintaining sense of smell and taste
- Synthesizing DNA
- Normal growth and development during pregnancy, childhood, and adolescence

Zinc Deficiency can Cause:
- Growth retardation.
- Hair loss.
- Diarrhea.
- Delayed sexual maturation.
- Impotence.
- Eye and skin lesions.
- Loss of appetite.
- Unwanted weight loss.
- Delayed healing of wounds.
- Taste abnormalities.
- Mental lethargy.
- Protein deficiency.
- Protein deficiency.
- Depletion of T & B cells in bone marrow and thyroid.

Zinc is found in:
- Red meat, poultry, beans, seafood, and vegetables.

Zinc for Growth

Zinc is called the "growth" mineral, but that doesn't mean it's just for kids. Zinc is essential at every stage of life for growth and development. Children, the elderly, and everyone in between need zinc.

Zinc is a component of the enzyme that triggers the synthesis of nucleic acids, the first step in the production of every cell. That's why zinc is important for people of all ages. The life span of cells is limited; new ones must constantly replace old ones. The faster this cell replacement is necessary, the more vital zinc becomes for the health of that particular tissue. Since zinc has its most profound influence on rapidly growing tissues, and its effect on reproduction is significant.

Other Functions

Zinc works with at least 200 different enzymes, including 80+ enzymes in the liver, which perform a wide variety of essential functions throughout the body. Without zinc, these enzymes may not work properly.

Zinc is also necessary to form tissues such as those in the skin, eyes, organs, and bones. Zinc promotes taste sensation and appetite. Zinc is a component of the hormone insulin, which regulates blood sugar levels. It is essential in normal glucose tolerance. The body's natural resistance to infection and inflammation can also depend on having enough zinc. Zinc is vital because it has the following functions: fights infection, essential for prostate health, helps sexual maturation, helps fetal development, decreases dental plaque formation, and supports healthy birth weight.

Zinc plays an important role in the health of the skin. Associated with wound healing, zinc is most critical in the latter part of the healing process, when the epidermal layers are healing. And zinc can be very effective in dealing with acne. A study of the role of oral zinc in the treatment of acne showed that a zinc supplement resulted in a decrease in acne scars in four weeks.

Food Sources for Zinc:

Certain foods may *interfere* with the body's absorption of zinc. Whole grains, nuts, and some vegetables contain a substance called "phytic acid," which unites with zinc, making it unavailable to the body.

The *best sources* of zinc are: eggs, fish, kelp, meat, legumes, pecans, pumpkin seeds, soy beans, lecithin, and sunflower seeds.

Herbs that contain zinc are: alfalfa, burdock root, cayenne, chamomile, chickweed, dandelion, fennel seed, milk thistle, nettle, parsley, rose hips, sage, sarsaparilla, and wild yam.

Zinc levels may be lowered by diarrhea, kidney disease, cirrhosis of the liver, diabetes, hard water, perspiration, or the intake of fiber.

When taking a supplement, it is best to take the recommended dose. Zinc gluconate is the most readily utilized form of zinc in a supplement form.

PART 3: HAPPY AND HEALTHY

Taste and see that the Lord is good, blessed is the man who trusts in Him.

Psalm 34:8 NKJ

Understanding your Health

HAPPY AND HEALTHY does not describe everyone today, but it does describe a great desire of many. In order to achieve this, we need to understand that we have a road block: chronic illness is enslaving us. Prevention is ideal, but many times illness is already upon us before we knew there were options.

If we take what we have learned about the nutritious foods given to us by God and make them a priority in our meal plans, then we will see changes in our health and happiness. Sometimes there are problems that have plagued our bodies for years and extra help and understanding are needed to overcome them. Part 3: Happy and Healthy will deal with specific health topics to assist you in obtaining a healthy body, healthy home, and healthy family. Therefore, your whole family will become happy as they are living in a healthy environment.

The teachings in this book are designed to give an overview on particular subjects and point to some simple changes that can be made to give your body what it needs to heal. The body is designed to heal itself, and we just need to better understand how it works in order to allow it to do its job in the best way possible. Please remember that these suggestions are not a replacement for the instructions your physician may suggest. Consult your physician for all medical advice treatment.

HEALTHY BODY

And may your spirit and soul and body be preserved complete.

1 Thessalonians 5:23

Developing the whole person

ONE OF MY favorite hymns is "Jesus is Tenderly Calling." I picture Jesus tenderly calling us to live our lives according to His will. God created us, and the Bible tells us that He knows our innermost being, and He knows what makes us happy. I picture Jesus encouraging us to put away all our worldly sins and follow His teachings. Yet many Christians neglect this plan and allow their lives to be dominated by sins that destroy their bodies, their mental health, their worship, their love for one another, and consequently, their happiness. It must be sad for Jesus to see His immaculate creation destroyed and suffering from poor health, mainly because of physical neglect. God wants us to be happy and to have the "abundant life." He tells us in the Bible that for us to be happy we have to learn to love God with all our hearts and with all our souls and with all our minds, and with all our strength, and to love our neighbor as ourselves. Hopefully from reading this book you will hear the call of Jesus tenderly pleading for you to develop your cells and life wholly according to His will so that you might better and longer serve Him.

Our Physical Health

"And Jesus increased in…stature." I picture Jesus as a highly conditioned person. I base my judgment on a study of his lifestyle. Jesus possessed a high oxygen intake, which was evident from the long distances he and his disciples traveled. There is evidence that Jesus once journeyed a distance of 120 miles in a three-day period (Mark 5–6).

In his early life, Jesus was a carpenter. His work required him to possess a great amount of strength. He didn't have power tools to aid him, and his tools were not sharpened by power-driven machines. It took strength and muscular endurance just to saw a board. We can see Jesus' strength and condition on the day he was beaten and crucified. Only a well-conditioned man could have survived the beating and torture that preceded the crucifixion.

God has created tremendous physical potential in the human body. When all areas of our health – digestion, immune system, brain, and heart – are physically balanced, we will reach greater potential.

AGING[48]

From birth to age twenty-five, we love the compliment "You look older." After twenty-five we typically run from those words. In fact, we do everything in our power to undo the pull of gravity on our bodies. Anti-wrinkle creams, permanent hair dyes, lotions that promise to remove ten years from our faces, exercise equipment to keep us toned as if we were thirty again. We are a nation caught up in the idea that we can look young forever. But is that possible?

Chronological aging is inevitable; day by day we grow older. In 365 days we are a year older. Biological aging is different. This aging process begins as soon as we stop growing in our late teens. Cell reproduction begins to slow and becomes less efficient, which starts the aging process. Once thought to be inevitable, like chronological aging, recent studies have shown that this process can be slowed by increasing the efficacy of cell repair and replication.

Our bodies are made up of millions of cells. These cells instruct the body on how to carry out virtually every miraculous function it performs. As we age, cells die and become damaged, thus increasing susceptibility to illness and disease.

The process of cellular aging is comprised of four mechanisms that lead to aging, disease, and eventually, death.

First Mechanism - DNA

Within each cell, at its center, is the nucleus. The nucleus houses the DNA of each cell, which carries important genetic information and defines the function of the cell. When all processes are working perfectly, the DNA is well protected and can be copied exactly when the cell divides, an essential function of cells. Our cells are attacked daily from the environment and our unhealthy lifestyles. This can damage or alter DNA structures. When DNA is under attack, the "database" included in the DNA is damaged and the function and longevity of the cell is compromised. Left unrepaired, these damaged cells still continue to replicate, creating millions of copies of damaged cells.

Second Mechanism – Genetic Regulators

The second mechanism of cellular aging comes from genetic regulators that contribute to age-related cellular deterioration. As the body ages, fewer cells are being repaired, and at the same time, more cells are dying.

Third Mechanism – Cellular Energy

The third mechanism of cellular aging is a decline in cellular energy production. Over time, free radicals are released by the mitochondria in the cells and deteriorate the mitochondria itself, which in turn reduces efficiency and releases even more free radicals. This effect is thought to be one of the major causes of cellular aging.

Fourth Mechanism – AGE Proteins

The fourth and final mechanism of cellular aging occurs with the accumulation of AGE (Advanced Glycation End products) proteins. These proteins are a byproduct of cell function and accumulate in a manner similar to that of plaque build-up in the arteries. As AGE proteins accrue, cell integrity and longevity is compromised.

To learn how to give your cells the ability to reverse the effects of aging, read about resveratrol in this manual. But without adding resveratrol as a supplement in your diet, the best way to prevent unnecessary aging is to be active with regular exercise outside in the fresh air and sunshine and eat a diet full of fresh fruits and vegetables. This should be a high fiber diet, including your own fresh-milled grain baked into a loaf of mouth-watering bread and drinking lots of purified water. Make each day special, and be grateful for all God has given you. The richest supplement you can add to increase your quality and longevity of life is the supplement of joy and gratitude.

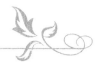

BRAIN HEALTH

Therefore, prepare your minds for action; be self-controlled; set your hope fully on the grace to be given you when Jesus Christ is revealed.

1 Peter 1:13

Better Foods Build Better Brains

Our digestive system is the UPS delivery guy for all the nutrients delivered to our bodies from the foods we consume. But there always seems to be one home that gets its packages delivered first, and our brain is that destination. Since a malfunctioning brain can take the rest of the body out of commission, the brain gets VIP status when the body distributes nutrients.

It has been proven in many homes and doctor offices for decades that there is a connection between how we eat and how we feel. Some foods help the brain work better, while other foods drag down the brain's performance. Three steps to help us are found in this verse in 1 Peter:

Prepare your minds for action (gird up the loins of your mind)

Be self-controlled (sober minded, sober in spirit)

Set your hope fully on the grace to be given you when Jesus Christ is revealed.

These foods will help you work toward these steps; applying discipline, your mind will be ready for action.

Brain Builders[50]

- Asparagus
- Bananas
- Broccoli
- Brussels sprouts
- Cheese, raw organic

- Avocados
- Lean beef, free range, farm
- Brown rice
- Cantaloupe
- Chicken, free range

- Collard greens
- Flaxseed, freshly ground
- Milk, raw
- Oranges
- Peas
- Romaine lettuce
- Soybeans, organic
- Tuna
- Wheat germ

- Eggs
- Legumes
- Oatmeal
- Peanut butter, organic
- Potatoes, sweet or new red
- Salmon
- Spinach
- Turkey
- Yogurt, organic

Brain Drainers

- Alcohol
- Colorings
- Soda
- Frostings
- Hydrogenated fats
- Nicotine
- White foods—bread, rice, vinegar, sugar, oils

- Artificial food
- Artificial sweeteners
- Corn syrup
- High-sugar drinks
- Junk sugars
- Overeating

Dr. Williams Sears, a practicing pediatrician, noticed differences in children based on the way they were fed in the home:

> Over my twenty-five years in pediatric practice, I have noticed a striking connection between how children are fed and how healthy they are. Mothers who consistently do not allow any unhealthy food to pollute the minds and bodies of their children seem to have healthier children. I have noticed that these children have fewer office visits and colds, and when they do come for periodic check-ups they seem more settled and better behaved. These "pure children" seem to get tagged with fewer labels, such as "A.D.D." or "learning disabled." Even when these children do warrant such tags, they seem to cope better with behavioral and learning differences and these seem less severe. These moms have made a believer out of me. I truly believe that there is a connection between how kids are fed and how they act and learn.[49]

Nutrition shows up quickly in children, but the same foods contributing to brain development in children works equally in adults. Everyone needs to make sure they are building healthy cells every day if they want to have a good mood and stay alert.

Specific Nutrition for the Brain

Our brains are sixty percent fat. That means the fat in our diet is extremely important. Fats are the major component of the brain cell membrane and the myelin sheath around each nerve. Healthy fats would include organic oils (fresh pressed), flaxseed, soy, and cold water fish. Supplements would be a good addition to every person's daily regime. Bad fats would include trans-fats, hydrogenated oils; partially hydrogenated oils, corn oil, and soy bean oil (if not organic).

Studies indicate that school children whose diets were supplemented with vitamins and minerals show improved learning and score higher on intelligence tests. Some of the recommended supplements and vitamins are:

- Multi Vitamin—age specific
- Vitamin C—the brain has its own vitamin C pump that draws extra vitamin C out of the blood and concentrates it in the brain.
- Vitamin B complex
- Iron
- Calcium
- Fiber: You could say, "An apple a day keeps the ADD away." Fiber does not contribute to the brain's nutrition directly, but the removal of toxic substances from the digestive tract allows the body to absorb the vital nutrients it needs to keep you alert.

BONE HEALTH

This will bring health to your body and nourishment to your bones.

Proverbs 3:8 NIV

GOD'S DESIGN OF bones is one of many intrinsic factors that could never have come from evolution. The value of our bones to our system is phenomenal yet, easily taken for granted. Indeed, the more we learn about our created design the more we understand how wonderfully made we are. Here are a few bony facts:

- The smallest bone in the human body is the stapes bone, which is located in the ear.
- There are 54 bones in your hands, including the wrists.
- The only bone fully grown at birth is located in the ear.
- The human face is made up of 14 bones.
- 4% of the total bone surface is going through a remodel continuously.
- Bones serve as a reservoir of calcium and other minerals – if the diet is insufficient of these nutrients it will pull from the bones.
- Humans are born with 300 bones in their bodies; however, when a person reaches adulthood, they only have 206 bones. This occurs because many of them join together to make a single bone.
- Gardening is said to be one of the best exercises for maintaining healthy bones.
- Although the outsides of a bone are hard, they are generally light and soft inside. They are about 75% water.
- Adult human bones account for 14% of the body's total weight.
- Your thigh bone is stronger than concrete.
- The strongest bone in your body is the femur (thighbone), and it's hollow!

Since your body is continually growing new bone, it is best to understand what makes our bones porous. Osteoporosis is not a disease of the older generation anymore. All ages are feeling the effects of this problem with the increased consumption of soft drinks. *Soft drinks make soft bones.* Exercise will help us build healthy bones.

OSTEOPOROSIS

Definition: Gradual loss of bone mass, resulting in fragile and brittle bones. Major cause is mal-absorption of calcium. It is a disease in which minerals are being depleted more rapidly than they can be replaced. Osteoporosis is sometimes called the "silent disease," since bone loss occurs without symptoms.

Goal: Build bone mass early in life, prior to the ages of 35–40. Then concentrate on maintaining that bone density. During childhood and early adolescence, it is critical that enough calcium is absorbed. Women past menopause lose the most bone mass: 1 in 2 women will have osteoporosis; however, some elderly men suffer the same conditions, 1 in 8. Seventy-eight percent of women over the age of 20 get less than 100% of the RDA for calcium. By the age of 20, the average woman has acquired 98% of her skeletal mass.

Good News: Bone density can be rebuilt. Following these recommendations for food and adding a good supplement with a quality calcium/magnesium supplement has been proven to reverse osteoporosis.

Risk Factors for Osteoporosis:
- Current cigarette smoking
- Heavy uses of alcohol
- Endurance athletes
- Eating disorders
- Junk food diets
- Avoiding weight-bearing exercises
- High intake of coffee, tea, colas,
- Taking anticoagulants, chemo, thyroid medication, diuretics, Cortisone medication, anti-seizure medications
- Post menopause and early menopause due to surgery
- Over age 65
- Anorexia
- Vitamin D deficiency
- Low testosterone levels
- An inactive lifestyle
- Being thin or small-framed

Also note that:

- The leading cause of lack of bone density is drinking sodas. The soda contains phosphates that cause the body to eliminate calcium, even if the calcium must be leached from the bones to do this. "Soft Drinks = Soft Bones"
- Milk and other dairy products are frequently spoken of as sources of dietary calcium, but studies have shown that consuming large quantities of dairy foods may actually end up robbing the body of calcium. Look for nondairy sources of calcium that you can incorporate into your diet. These sources will provide variety and give you enough calcium to build up the necessary bone density to prevent or slow the progression of osteoporosis.

Methods of increasing bone density:
- Diet rich in calcium; magnesium; phosphorus; vitamins D, C, and K; and adding a good quality soy protein. See "Calcium & Magnesium."
- Vitamin C and protein are needed for collagen formation. This matrix helps the bone tissue to form. See "Vitamin C" and "Protein."
- The mineral boron improves calcium absorption by 40%. Some great food sources include almonds, Brazil nuts, hazelnuts, figs, prunes, apples, grapes, dates, raisins, pears, peaches, soybeans, honey, and molasses.
- Pineapples protect strong bones because they contain manganese. Alfalfa also has a good amount of manganese.
- Spend time outside every day. Fifteen minutes a day in the sun will help. The sun's ultraviolet radiation on our skin produces vitamin D, which is necessary for calcium absorption. Sun block will block the absorption.
- Weight-bearing exercise. As the muscles and tendons pull and push on the bone, these forces promote more healthy bone formation.
- Supplement with a well-balanced calcium magnesium product. See "Calcium Magnesium."

Physical Exercise

For the person seeking health, exercise is as important as nutrition or sleep. So, are you ready for a fitness program? How do you view your body? Is it treasured as a gift? Or is it just available to use at your disposal? How we care for our bodies reflect our views of God.

God has gifted us with a "fearfully and wonderfully made" (see Psalm 139) temple that is designed to perfectly glorify Him. In the ancient days, the glory of the God of Israel dwelt within the sanctuary of the temple, and meticulous care was taken to honor His throne. Do we take that same care of our physical temple today (see 1 Cor. 6:19–20)? There is a holy call to worship our Creator by offering our bodies as living sacrifices in gratitude for the price He paid for us (Romans 12:1).

As Christians we cannot fulfill the planned purpose of God if we are unhealthy due to neglecting our bodies. God has ordained us as stewards, and we cannot fully develop spiritually until we have developed physically.

So how do we develop physically? We've learned about eating and resting properly, but the other component to a healthy lifestyle involves exercise and movement. Exercise is important for the following reasons:

- An increased general feeling of health and well being
- Getting tired less easily
- Prevention, delay, or a great ability to withstand and recover from heart problems and other degenerative diseases
- Controlled body weight
- Improved posture and appearance
- Relief of tension and/or stress
- Prevention of lower back pain
- Delayed aging process
- Delayed aging of brain cells
- Improved neuromuscular skill and physical performance
- Clearer thinking
- Better digestion and bowel movement
- Improved functioning of the internal organs

The improvements to our health and the personal testimony give us an insight to the power of this discipline of exercise. Who do you know who could benefit from adding five minutes of exercise or stretching into their daily lives?

Sometimes it's difficult to find motivation to exercise. But changing our attitudes and mindsets is essential in order to find inspiration. Some ways to think positively:

- Focus on the benefits of exercise: increased energy, mental focus, and self-esteem; weight loss, staving off disease, and longer life.
- Set goals.
- Look for improvements: a faster mile, a few more reps, or one less dress size.
- Join your foodie friend or find a buddy.
- Do something you like.
- Spend time with God on a run, bike ride, etc.

Getting Started

There are many different ways to exercise, and a great variety of goals can be achieved. The most important forms of exercise are those targeting the cardiovascular system, which refers specifically to the heart and blood vessels, but benefits every system in the body. You can do other forms of exercise after you are fit from a cardiovascular standpoint, but it would be foolish to do them in lieu of other exercises.

If your goal is to lose weight, the same exercises contributing cardiovascular fitness also are best for weight loss. Some people think to lose fat from a certain part of the body, you exercise that part. For instance, if someone wants to lose belly fat, they do crunches. The fact is that your body has a blueprint it follows on where to store fat. Unfortunately, we can't change! The only way to get rid of fat is to burn more calories than you consume. Usually a one-two punch of restricting intake and increasing the burn rate through exercise works the best. If we want to burn more calories, we exercise the biggest muscles in our bodies, which are in our legs, not the tiny muscles found around our abdomen. As you burn calories through exercise, your body takes off fat according to the blueprint.

No one is excused from exercising. Even those who are unable to walk can exercise their arms and chest muscles. If you have not exercised in the last several years, there are several tips for getting started. But the most important thing to remember is the need to move.

Cardiovascular and Aerobic Fitness

Note: It is helpful to understand cardiovascular health and target heart rate when doing an exercise program.

Cardiovascular workouts are the most important of any fitness regime because they strengthen the heart, blood, blood vessels, and lungs. Circulatory disease affects the heart and lungs and is the leading cause of death in the world. Maintaining cardiovascular fitness prevents these diseases in most cases.

Cardio workouts are intense sessions that raise your heart rate to receive training benefits. You can elevate heart rate by walking briskly, running, swimming, cycling, and playing vigorous sports. To determine your target heart rate to set as your goal during exercise:

- Subtract your age from 220. This is your maximum heart rate.
- Prior to exercise, count your heart rate (pulse) for one minute (this will be your resting heart rate), and subtract that number from your maximum heart rate.
- Multiply the difference by 0.7 if you have been exercising consistently and by 0.6 if you haven't exercised in months or are over fifty years old.
- Add your resting heart rate again to get your aerobic threshold:
- 220 - _____age= _____ (maximum heart rate)

    -_____ (resting heart rate)

    =_____ x 0.7 (or 0.6)

    =_____ + resting heart rate

    =_____ desired working heart rate or aerobic threshold.

If you are just starting an exercise program, start slowly and train at around 70 to 60% of your aerobic threshold. Duration of exercise should mirror what your fitness level is. If you can only do five or ten minutes of exercise at first, that's all right. Do what you can. Your body will adjust as you get stronger, and you will be able to handle more in a few weeks. If you are fit, you should be exercising longer. The key is consistency; make an effort to exercise at least three times a week, preferably four to six times. Once five minutes is no longer a struggle, increase your time by five minutes every week until you are up to twenty minutes. Set aside a time of day you prefer, and stick to your schedule.

If you have been inactive for four weeks or longer, start a walking program to slowly develop your leg muscles. For older adults or those with a low level of cardiovascular fitness, walking provides enough physical stress to increase cardiovascular fitness.

Check out these important things to remember:

- Get a medical examination before starting an exercise program.
- Always warm up before exercising.
- Cool down after exercising.
- Exercise within your tolerance.
- Progress slowly.
- Get adequate rest and nutrition.
- Exercise regularly.
- Wear proper shoes.
- Exercise cautiously in hot weather.
- Dress appropriately in cold conditions.

Strength Training

Strengthen the weak hands, and make firm the feeble knees.

Isaiah 35:3 RSV

Weight training, if done properly, will not make you look like Arnold Schwarzenegger or break feeble bones. There are over six hundred muscles, and research has shown that muscles will degenerate if they are not constantly used and strengthened. Training the muscles will help correct posture, lower back pain, and neck joint disorders; build muscular balance, endurance, and strength; and prevent injuries when exercising. Two thirty to sixty minute workouts per week should be sufficient for building the muscles.

Don't forget to build your abdominals. Our core muscles protect our lower back and are the stabilization to every movement we make. It's important to build these muscles in order to increase strength, agility, power, and speed.

If you've never done weight training before, I suggest finding a book at the library that shows different exercises for specific muscles and the proper form to do them. It may also be helpful to find a personal trainer who will supervise your workout sessions. When developing a program, you will want to include all five types of muscular contractions and movements:

1. **Flexion:** bending or decreasing the angle between two bones; for example, bringing the forearm to the shoulder

2. **Extension:** increasing the angle between two bones, as in returning the forearm to its original straight position

3. **Abduction:** moving the bone away from the midline of the body (the invisible line divides the body into right and left halves); for example, raising the arm out to the side of the body

4. **Adduction:** moving the bone towards the midline of the body; for example, returning the arm to the side

5. **Circumduction:** moving in all planes; for example, rotating the arms in circles

Stretching

Stretching is essential for maintaining flexibility, reducing muscle soreness, and preventing injury. Take at least ten minutes each day to stretch out all of your main muscle groups; this will help keep you relaxed and limber. Stretching in the morning will make you ready for the day. Some of these stretches can be done while sitting at a desk. Here is an example of an easy stretching routine:

- **Head:** Gently roll your neck in a circle several times. Switch directions.
- **Neck:** Place your right hand over your head and onto the left ear. Gently pull with your hand and tilt your head towards the right. Repeat on the opposite side.
- **Triceps:** Lift one arm in the air, bend your elbow, and place the arm behind your head. Place the other hand on the bent elbow, stretching out the back of the arm. Repeat on the opposite side.
- **Shoulders:** Clasp your hands together, out in front of you. Roll the palms outward while hunching over to stretch out the shoulders.
- **Sides:** Lift your right arm in air; place your left hand on your hip. Bend over to your left, stretching out the right side. Repeat on the left side.
- **Hips:** Stand with your feet farther than shoulder width apart. Bend at the knees into a deep plié, placing your hands on the tops of the thighs for support. Feel the stretch in the inner thigh and groin area.
- **Hamstrings:** Place feet together, step the right foot out about two feet. Lean forward

at the waist, keeping the back straight. Feel the back of the leg stretch. Repeat on the left side.

- **Quadriceps:** Bend your right leg back behind you and grab the foot with your right hand. Feel the front of the thigh stretch. Repeat on the other side.
- **Calf:** Stand on the edge of a stair, place your foot so your heel is off of the stair. Gently push your heel down to stretch the back of the calf. Repeat on the other side.

Please keep in mind that whatever exercise you choose to do will only be effective if you stick with it. The first couple of months are the most crucial. Especially at the very beginning, your body will complain, your schedule will resist, and you will think of a thousand reasons not to continue. If you persevere, the reward of a gift of better health awaits you. You will sleep better. You will look better and feel better—not just physically, but emotionally as well. Exercise not only puts the physical benefits back into our lives, but also the emotional benefits. Exercise gives us time to think. If we do it with a spouse or friend, it gives us a time for healthy, informal interaction with others.

Make every day an opportunity to move purposefully and intensely. We draw close to Jesus by appreciating who He has created us to be and discovering the unique capabilities of our bodies. Remember, we are accountable to God for the way we control our bodies.

DIGESTION

OVER FIFTY MILLION visits to the doctor each year are due to problems in the digestive system. God's intricate architecture of the GI (gastro intestinal) tract makes it sensitive and responsive to conditions in its environment. Knowing what the optimal conditions are will help you to promote the best functions of the system.

One indispensible condition is good health of the digestive tract itself. This health is affected by such factors of lifestyle as sleep, diet, obesity, exercise, and state of mind. Adequate sleep allows for repair, maintenance of tissues, and removal of wastes that might impair efficient functioning. Exercise promotes healthy muscle tone. A good mental state profoundly affects digestion and absorption; you should be relaxed and tranquil (not asleep) at mealtimes.

Another factor is the kind of meals you eat. Among the characteristics of meals that promote optimal absorption of nutrients are balance, variety, adequacy, and moderation. Balance means having neither too much nor too little of anything. For example, some fat is needed; fat slows intestinal motility, permitting time for absorption of some of the nutrients that are slow to be absorbed. Balance also includes fiber. Too little fiber means the digestive tract will be sluggish and toxic. Too much fiber means the nutrients will not be given time to be absorbed. Variety is important since there is no one food that gives us everything we need. Instead, a balanced diet with a variety of vegetables, fiber-rich foods, fruits, and grains will keep us going for a long time.

As for adequacy, it could be said that every nutrient depends on every other. All the nutrients work together, and all are present in the cells of a healthy digestive tract. To maintain health and promote the functions of the GI tract, you should make balance, variety, adequacy, and moderation features of every day's menus.

Energizing Enzymes:

Nutrition cannot be explained without describing the role enzymes play. Enzymes are like the spark plugs to your car; without them, you don't go anywhere. Enzymes are protein chemicals that carry a vital energy factor needed for every chemical action and reaction that occurs in our bodies. There are approximately 20,000 different enzymes found in the human cell. These enzymes can combine with vitamins and minerals to form nearly 100,000 various chemicals (that we know of today) that enable us to see, feel, move, digest food, and think.

Every cell in the body depends on certain enzymes, that spark plug. All enzymes are specific in their duties. A protein digestive enzyme will not digest fat; a fat enzyme will not digest a starch. Each enzyme has a specific function in the body.

When we eat raw foods, their enzyme activity can begin at the very moment the plant cell walls are ruptured by chewing. The saliva also contains enzymes, which begin to break down the food. After swallowing, digestive function continues in the food enzymes section of the stomach for thirty minutes to one hour.

The body should manufacture a supply of enzymes, but it can and also should obtain enzymes from food. With the increase of processed and highly cooked foods, our bodies have greatly decreased the amount of enzymes they make. It is necessary to understand that enzymes are sensitive to heat, and even low to moderate heat destroys most enzymes in food. To obtain enzymes from your diet, you must eat raw foods. Eating raw foods along with taking a supplement helps prevent depletion of the body's own enzymes and thereby reduces the stress on the body.

Enzymes are very powerful and necessary for digestion and other body reactions, but they cannot act alone. They require a large amount of coenzymes to be fully active. These coenzymes come from vitamins and minerals such as B-complex, vitamin C, vitamin E, and zinc.

When choosing an enzyme supplement, choose a plant-based one that contains all of the major enzyme groups, amylase, protease, and lipase. It is not necessary to take a different enzyme product for every digestive condition. There are supplements available that cover all areas. Some health related supplements will include enzymes to allow the product to work better.

Research has shown that as we grow older, the body's ability to produce enzymes decreases. This is the time that many elderly people have mal-absorption of nutrients and tissue breakdown and chronic health conditions increase. Taking supplemental enzymes can help to ensure that you continue to get the full nutritional value from your foods. Some sources state that enzyme supplementation is vital for elderly people.

Digestion and Enzymes

Basics:

- Slow down; take time to chew your food. This allows the enzymes in your saliva to begin to break down the food as you are chewing.
- Sit while eating; this makes it easier on your body and creates a more relaxed system to handle the digestion.
- Do not overeat; it takes about twenty minutes for your brain to receive a signal that you are full. Eating fast just delays that signal; therefore, you overeat.
- Take a break; placing the demand on your body to continually digest food depletes your reservoir of digestive enzymes. Eating late at night can continue to deplete your source of enzymes and increase "wear and tear" on your body. Consider fasting for a meal every once in a while to replenish your enzymes.
- Include zinc and protein; including zinc and protein in your daily diet will help your body manufacture digestive enzymes.
- Water: Drinking water thirty minutes before a meal and two hours after a meal will increase the effectiveness of the enzymes in your body for digestion. Eliminating water (or other drinks) during the meal will prevent the enzymes from being diluted, thereby decreasing their ability to work.
- Yogurt and probiotics restore the proper balance of good bacteria in your digestive tract will decrease digestive disorders. You can read about this under the title "Probiotics and Yogurt."
- Natural forms of digestive aids:

  - Alfalfa—as a supplement or as a sprout on your salad or sandwich
  - Plant-based digestive aid—this comes in the form of a supplement and should cover all types of enzymes (protein, carbohydrates, dairy, legumes, etc. in one tablet). Take this each day with your biggest meal. Some people who have had their gallbladder removed may need this with each meal.
  - Pineapple/ Papaya—excellent to have in the diet each week (fresh).
  - Ginger—½–1 teaspoon freshly ground ginger to a cup of water, let it steep for ten minutes, strain ginger, and then drink. You can also add ginger to your bean recipe to help eliminate the gas-producing effect.

- Stress: It is critical to reduce the stress in your life. Take time to enjoy your meals and have music playing the background that is comforting—that is, unless you have a table of kids to enjoy listening to.
- Fiber: Increase your fiber until you are having a minimum of one bowel movement daily.

Leaky Gut Syndrome

As many as 20 – 30 years before signs and symptoms become detectable, people have a steady decline in body function. Leaky Gut Syndrome is another name for Increased Intestinal Permeability. It includes a large variety of illnesses and symptoms. It is not a disease in itself. As you see in the list of associated conditions (below), it doesn't seem that they are related; but they are. People who have any of these conditions usually also have a leaky gut. The list below seems to grow each year as the medical profession learns more about this illness and the full understanding of digestion. All of the symptoms can arise from a variety of causes, but leaky gut may underlie more classic diagnosis.

Common Clinical Conditions Associated with Increased Intestinal Permeability:

- Acne
- AIDS
- Allergic disorders
- Arthritis/ inflammation/ joint disease
- Autoimmune diseases
- Chemotherapy (need for)
- Chronic Fatigue Syndrome
- Cystic fibrous
- Eczema
- Environmental illness
- Giardiasis
- Hives
- Inflammatory bowel disease
- Irritable bowel syndrome
- Mal-absorbtion
- Multiple chemical sensitivities
- Pancreatic insufficiency
- Reiter's syndrome
- Schizophrenia
- Thermal injury
- Ulcerative colitis
- Aging
- Alcoholism
- Ankylosing Spondylitis
- Asthma
- Celiac disease
- Childhood hyperactivity
- Crohn's disease
- Digestive issues
- Endotoxemia
- Food allergies/ sensitivities
- HIV positive
- Inflammation
- Intestinal infections
- Liver dysfunction
- Migraines
- NSAID enteropathy
- Psoriasis
- Rheumatoid Arthritis
- Systemic Lupus
- Trauma

Symptoms Associated with Leaky Gut Syndrome:

- Abdominal pain
- Anxiety
- Bed wetting
- Chronic joint pain
- Aggressive behavior
- Asthma
- Bloating
- Chronic muscle pain

- confusion
- Diarrhea
- Fevers of unknown origin
- Gas
- Mood Swings
- Poor immunity
- Poor memory
- Recurrent bladder infections
- Skin rashes and other skin issues

- Constipation
- Fatigue/ malaise
- Fuzzy thinking
- Indigestion
- Nervousness
- Poor exercise tolerance
- Primary Bladder infections
- Recurrent vaginal infections
- Shortness of breath

The Digestive System and Leaky Gut:

The digestive system handles everything that enters our mouths until it leaves our bodies. Two-thirds of our immune system is around the digestive system. This system decides whether food is a friend or foe. Our health comes down to the health of this one system and its ability to communicate with the rest of the body.

It is a system that needs great care and attention. Every three to five days it repairs and replaces itself. This is important to understand as we look for improving its functions.

The intestine is constantly being exposed to toxins, irritants, foods, and microbes. The intestinal tract provides a barrier between the outside world and what actually gets absorbed into our bodies. When the intestinal barrier becomes inflamed or breached, microbes and foreign substances gain entrance into us and can create any sort of trouble imaginable. When this happens, over a period of time we begin to suffer any number of the symptoms in the previous lists.

Nutritious foods are the right place to start for a healthy body, but some people may still have a digestive disorder due to the lack of enzymes in their bodies to help break down and absorb the nutrients in foods. Leaky gut is primarily an absorption problem—too many substances are allowed to pass from the intestinal lining into the blood stream.

Causes for Leaky Gut:

- Alcohol
- Cancer therapies
- Chronic Stress
- GMO foods
- Pain medications—long term use
- Steroid Medications
- Toxic overload/ environment contaminants (household cleaners, personal care items)

- Antibiotics
- Candida
- Food sensitivities*
- Lack of good bacteria
- Poor food choices – fast food diet
- Sugar

Sign of food allergies in children: ADD, behavior problems, learning problems, and recurring ear infections. Food allergies are typically caused by leaky gut syndrome. The good news is that the digestive system is designed to repair itself.

Restoring Your Digestive System

1) *Chew your food carefully.* This is the beginning of digestion—chewing increases the surface area of your food, while the saliva contains digestive enzymes that begin the process of digesting of carbohydrates and fats.

2) *Avoid food that causes allergic reactions.* *If you are not sure you are allergic to a food or food group, abstain from that group for 1–2 weeks and see if the symptoms lessen. Try this with other food groups through a rotation diet.

3) *Probiotics/prebiotics*—this supplement is needed by most people to increase the good bacteria in their systems, along with FOS or inulin.

4) *Enzymes*—take an enzyme product that helps your body break down the foods. (See resource section.)

5) *Antioxidants*—Vitamin E, Carotenoids, Flavonoids, CoQ10, Vitamin C

6) Fresh fruits and vegetables

7) Multi-Vitamin

8) B-complex

9) Zinc

*Almost any food can cause a reaction. When you try to eliminate foods, you are left with enormous cravings for these foods, and symptoms worsen before they improve. This can take 7–10 days to get through this stage.

How to Remove the Toxins

Fruit and vegetable cleansing—this is gentle but effective. Eat all you want of fruits, vegetables, rice, and olive oil for seven to ten days. If you want to continue after this time, you can add fish, poultry, legumes, nuts, and seeds. If constipation becomes a problem, then add flax seed, freshly ground, or a fiber product with psyllium seeds. Drink lots of purified water plus herbal teas if you want some flavor.

Reduce Your Exposure to Toxins.

There are environmental toxins that you are exposed to every day that you have no control over, such as exhaust fumes, secondhand cigarette smoke, and air pollution. But there are steps you can take to benefit your health:

- Avoid Medications—especially over the counter NSAID.
- Avoid Alcohol.
- Buy organic foods.
- Reduce or eliminate food additives. The average person consumes fourteen pounds each year of these, including colorings, flavorings, and preservatives.
- Avoid herbicides and pesticides.
- Use natural cleaning products—there are a few brands that clean better than regular cleaners and are safe for the environment and your family and will even save you money.

Rules for a Lifetime of Healthful Eating
- Eat local foods in season.
- Life in foods gives us life.
- Plan ahead and carry food with you to avoid getting hungry while you are out.
- Eat when you are hungry; stop when you are satisfied.
- Avoid high-calorie, low-nutrient foods.
- Choose organically grown whenever possible.
- Eat as many fruits and veggies as possible.
- Drink clean water.
- Eat lots of fiber.
- Respect your own body's uniqueness.
- Relax while eating.
- Learn to handle stress before it handles you.
- Exercise.

Hiatal Hernia/ Esophageal Reflux/ Acid Reflux/ Heartburn/ Sour Stomach
- Concentrate on all of the basics mentioned in regards to digestion and enzymes.
- Apple Cider Vinegar: adding either 1 teaspoon or up to tablespoon in water before eating is helpful for many people.
- Avoid Common Offenders—they relax the sphincter muscle, causing it to open and allow stomach acid to backwash or increase acidity of stomach juices.
- Avoid eating 4-5 hours before bedtime.
- Lose weight.
- Increase fiber and avoid large fat meals.

a. chocolate	b. coffee/tea
c. alcohol	d. carbonated drinks/soda
e. sugar	f. fats

g. onions

h. citrus

i. dairy (*milk is #1 problem*)

j. spicy foods

This list is different for each person. After beginning a healthy diet, you may find these symptoms disappearing in a very short time.

For us, Steve's symptoms were gone in three days after following a very healthy diet and using a fiber supplement. His symptoms have not returned since 2004! We discovered ice cream was the main culprit. He can still have this food, but in moderation—just as it says in Scripture.

Colon and Colon Therapy

Today, Americans are suffering from colon problems that affect over 90% of the population. The problems associated with the colon lead to a multitude of other problems throughout the body. Over 79% of our immune systems are located near our colons and digestive tracts. Most of these problems are labeled diseases of one type or another and are given specific names. However, regardless of their labels, most of these specific diseases come directly from impactions, miscellaneous debris, or toxic materials that are formed in the colon and generate toxins throughout the rest of the body—a direct cause of many of the diseases of mankind.

Dr. George C. Crile, head of the Crile Clinic in Cleveland and one of the world's greatest surgeons, said, "There is no natural death. All deaths that come from so-called natural causes are merely the end point of progressive acid saturation. Many people go so far as to consider that sickness and disease are just a 'cross' or an element which God gave them to bear here on this earth. However, if they would take care of their body and cleanse their colon and intestines, their problems would be pretty much eliminated and they could eliminate their 'cross' by proper diet, proper exercise, and in general, proper living."[51]

As we examine the functions of the body and of the colon, it seems only normal and reasonable that if we can prevent toxins from building up in the system and help the body to cleanse and heal itself, we can eliminate nearly all of the diseases generated by these toxins.

Every cell of the body needs not only to be cleansed but also to be nourished. Every cell of the body tends to add to or subtract from the overall health of the system. There is no single, individual problem in the body that every part of the body is not indirectly or directly related to. Every part of the body is affected by the nervous system, the lymphatic system, and all the other systems of the entire body. Upon close observation, we will find that there is actually only one disease, and that is deficient emptying or deficient cleansing of the system. The name of the disease depends upon where the poisons settle and where they are primarily located. Thus, from these same toxins we can have:

- Arthritis
- Cancer
- Diverticulitis
- Indigestion
- Liver problems
- Neuritis
- Rheumatism

- Autoimmune disorders
- Depression
- Gallbladder problems
- Kidney problems
- Nausea
- Obesity
- Sciatica

All of these come from an accumulation of mucous and a re-absorption of toxins and other debris within the system.

Whenever we develop weak cells, it is almost always due to the fact that the body has been deficient in the materials needed to keep the cells rebuilt and functioning properly. Thus, we can determine that most problems within the colon itself are caused from deficiency in the diet and from deficiency in nourishment within the system itself.

COMPLICATED CONSTIPATION

Constipation is one of America's major problems. It also contributes to many of our health problems. Constipation is a problem and is a result of our hurried way of eating, eating processed foods, and eating foods that our bodies do not know how to handle well and that it cannot push through the system as well as it should.

The collection of the materials in the body can cause the bowels to extend and cause large bowel obstruction and large bowel pockets that tend to cause disease throughout the system. If we can eliminate constipation and keep our colon clean, we can eliminate many of the other problems that are inherent in the body due to the poor digesting problems.

The large intestine is capable of spasms, strictures, impactions, and blocks all at the same time.

Causes of Constipation:
- Diet—too much processed food, refined sugar, refined grains, and dairy
- Medications—pain medications, anti-depressants, antacids that contain aluminum, diuretics, and antibiotics
- Lack of exercise—exercise stimulates lymphatic flow, which helps create normal peristalsis
- Travel or change in routine
- Tension

Signs of Good Elimination:
- Stool color—medium brown, unless eating certain foods changes this temporarily
- Consistency and length—1½ inches in diameter (the size of a clean, healthy colon), total for the day should be 24 inches and approximately 2 pounds. Now you need a ruler and scale in the bathroom☺.
- Floater or Sinker?—Normal, healthy stool leaves the body easily and gently settles in the water. If there is not enough fiber in the diet, it may plummet to the bottom of the toilet. "Floaters" may be a sign of inadequate fiber or too much undigested fat.
- 2–3 times a day—At least one bowel movement per day. Your goal should be 2–3 times per day, depending on food intake.

Simple Steps to Achieve Daily Elimination
- Water/hydration—the best way to stimulate peristalsis is through proper hydration of the colon. Constipation is often caused by dehydration.
- Supplement with calcium/magnesium tablets—magnesium is a gentle mineral that brings water into the colon.
- Fiber is the important key. The colon requires bulk for it to move 2–3 times per day. Read about fiber in the nutrition chapter of this manual.
- Flax Seed—this will add to the fiber intake and contribute to a healthy colon.
- Lubrication—Oils help provide smooth and gentle elimination. These include essential fatty acids, such as oils in flaxseed, cold water fish, or supplements like EPA or GLA.
- Exercise

Laxative Pitfalls
Probably the greatest single cause of constipation is the widespread use of laxatives and synthetic colon therapies. They are all harmful when taken daily for any length of time, because a good many of these laxatives contain dangerous and harmful drugs like phenolphthalein and belladonna, which are all very harmful to the system. Laxatives have never cured a single case of constipation. They actually create cases of chronic constipation.

Mineral oil is not absorbed by the bowel, as are other laxatives, but it acts by gravity, forcing itself by its own weight down the gastrointestinal tract and greasing it. This grease disturbs digestion by preventing the digestive juices from getting to the food, and it prevents absorption of the lining in the intestinal wall.

Various herbal formulas will increase the peristaltic action of the colon to help it function better. As it does this, it will actually increase the peristaltic action and help the body to take over its functions. Many of the herbs that have been created for this purpose by God will help this process.

Herbs to Help Detoxify the Body and Reduce Constipation:
- Alfalfa leaf
- Anise seed
- Blue malva flower
- Buckthorn bark
- Culvers root
- Fennel seed
- Licorice root
- Rhubarb root
- Senna leaf

A combination of these herbs will contribute to a healthy colon, and you will never have to worry about the results from a colonoscopy again!

Remember, you are only as healthy as your colon. It can be a cesspool of toxins poisoning your system, or it can be a garden where the vitality of life flows to your entire being, creating a state of pure health and vitality for a lifetime of vibrant living.

Worms and Parasites

Probably one of the most common of all digestive problems is caused by worms and parasites. Certain practitioners put various labels on these different categories.

Parasites enter our bodies through our own contaminated hands when we handle things polluted by the eggs or the larva and from the foods we ingest. Meat is probably one of the biggest contributors of parasites to the body. Some other ways of getting parasites is through handling animals and pets—dogs, cats, birds, and almost every creature that lives outside can be carriers.

Symptoms of Worms:
- Not being able to sleep easily at night
- Gritting of the teeth during sleep and even when awake
- Constant coughs
- Some types of acne and eczema

In Order to Get Rid of Parasites

First you must find and remove the cause. Make every step to improve the daily living environment. Constipation contributes to the parasite problem. One suggestion to get rid of parasites is to fast on fruit or fruit juice for several days, along with eating pumpkin seeds—½ –1 pound per day. Also drink freely of fennel seed tea or senna seed tea or (this is true) wormwood tea. There are many herbal teas that tend to eliminate and get rid of parasites. Garlic will also kill parasites.

Celiac Disease and Gluten Intolerance

Celiac disease, which affects less than 1% of Americans, is caused by the body's inability to properly digest foods containing a particular protein component of gluten, known as gliadin. Gluten is the naturally occurring protein of most grains, particularly wheat. When grain, such as wheat, is milled the bran and germ are removed leaving the white flour which is then bleached and bromated. For the past 100 years the American diet has been increasing in nutrient empty processed foods. Add to this problem the addition of GMO foods in the late 1990's and you have a recipe for disaster in the digestive system.

Even though the consumption of wheat has dropped dramatically in the last 40 years the increase in GMO foods has risen to over 80% of all foods purchased in the grocery store. Many authorities have come to the conclusion gluten is the blame but fail to look beyond their pen to see the facts that the increase in GMO foods more correlates to the increase in digestive issues than the decrease in wheat consumption.

Since GMO foods are proven to be destructive to the lining of the digestive tract this is the precursor to the gluten intolerance and hence celiac disease. The sad conclusion is the disruption in God's design for foods is that those with celiac can no longer enjoy the 'bread of life' as mentioned in Scripture numerous times.

Gluten intolerance is not a permanent condition. Even wheat allergy is temporary. Those suffering from this condition should consider going gluten free for 3 months to 2 years. During that time the addition of a multi vitamin, iron, magnesium and zinc supplementation will help the digestive system to heal. Then the person can introduce wheat bread ONLY if they mill the grains themselves and make their own bread. Because of the pain associated with gluten sensitivity it is not recommended to ever eat processed grains again.

Three ingredients necessary for the development of Celiac disease are the right genetics plus gluten plus a leaky gut. This is important to understand since two of the three can be controlled by you. Eating whole grains that you mill yourself make the gluten able to be processed with the added nutrients God designed in the grain. Leaky gut can also be controlled by you. Read more about this in this Manual.

Two ingredients necessary for the development of gluten intolerance is leaky gut and gluten. Both of which you can control for the most part if you are a very smart shopper and desire to make your own foods.

Common Symptoms:
- Abdominal pain, distention, gas, indigestion
- Constipation or diarrhea
- Other food allergies, such as to milk
- Malnutrition
- Nausea and vomiting
- Weight loss or gain

Related Complications:
- Anemia
- Bone and joint pain
- Dermatitis Herpetiformis or other skin disorders
- Fatigue
- Growth delay in children
- Mood swings
- Osteoporosis
- Steatorrhea (gray or tan, fatty, greasy, foul-smelling stools that float)

The only treatment for celiac is a life-long adherence to a gluten-free diet, which allows the intestines to heal. You must carefully read all food, medication, supplements, personal care products and drink labels to find hidden sources of gluten. Hydrolyzed/textured vegetable protein, modified food starch, soy sauce, grain vinegars, binders, fillers, gravies, lunch meats, beer, mustard, ketchup, nondairy creamer, white vinegar, and seasonings can all be contaminated, so it's important to check before eating. Some alternatives include: rice, corn, soy, potato, tapioca, beans, garfava, sorghum, quinoa, millet, buckwheat, arrowroot, amaranth, teff, montina, flax, and nut flours.

Lifestyle Tips:
- Learn to read labels carefully. This is important to maintain good health.
- Join a local support group.
- Learn to cook.
- When eating out, talk to the server about your needs and don't be shy about inquiries.
- Exercise, even as simple as walking, should be incorporated into your lifestyle.
- Eat fresh vegetables, legumes, fruits, organic lean meats, and dairy products. Most foods in their natural state are gluten-free. Packaged foods are less likely to be safe. If you follow the principles for God's design, then it should be easy to go gluten-free!
- Avoid processed gluten-free products. The healthiest way to be gluten free is to

control everything you eat. You do the cooking, baking, etc. Eating processed foods such as gluten-free packaged foods is leading to other problems with the increased amount of flavor enhancers, preservatives and additives to make these foods palatable.

Gluten Intolerance vs. Celiac Disease:

Gluten intolerance is a broad term that includes all kinds of sensitivity to gluten. A small proportion of gluten intolerant people will test positive to Celiac Disease; however, these people still benefit from a gluten-free diet. Most gluten sensitive people return negative or inconclusive results upon Celiac testing. It's important to follow an elimination diet and then introduce one new food at a time while focusing on changes in the body.

Lactose Intolerance

Lactose Intolerance is different from a milk allergy. Someone with an allergy has an immune system response to one or more of milk's proteins. Lactose Intolerance is the inability to digest lactose, a type of milk sugar. Lactose is a "double" sugar made from linked glucose and galactose. Double sugars are too large to be absorbed, so they must be split by an enzyme called lactase. Everyone is born producing enough lactase; however, by the age of five most bodies stop producing the lactase enzyme. Without the enzyme present, the food ferments and bacteria feed on the sugar, producing gas and bloating. Other symptoms include:

- Abdominal cramps, bloating
- Diarrhea
- Floating or foul-smelling stools
- Gas
- Malnutrition
- Weight Loss
- Nausea

Some adults, especially those of European ancestry, continue to produce enough lactase. However, about 75% of the world's adults—Asians, Africans, Middle Easterners, and Native Americans—do not make much or any lactase.[1] The amount of dairy your body can handle is an individual matter that depends on what bacteria is in your body and how much lactase you produce. People who suffer from lactose intolerance can often tolerate yogurt and hard cheeses in small doses, because the healthy bacteria used to produce these foods feed on the lactose sugar. You can also try Lactaid or an enzyme supplement product that will allow you to eat dairy foods.

This disease, along with Celiac, seems to put the blame on the food, in this case, dairy, instead of the processing. When raw milk is studied, it is proven to include the enzyme lactase naturally for everyone to be able to enjoy dairy foods. Read more about raw milk in the Nutrition section under "Milk."

Dairy alternatives:
- Soy milk – only organic, cheese, sour cream, cream cheese, pudding, ice cream, butter
- Almond milk
- Rice milk, yogurt
- Hemp milk
- Coconut milk, yogurt
- Goat's milk
- Lactose-free dairy milk.

Be sure to look for items labeled "vegan," as you can be assured that they will not contain dairy products. And don't overdo on the processed foods, especially soy.

Remember, it's important to make sure you're getting enough calcium through enriched dairy alternatives, a vitamin, or from calcium-rich vegetables.

Diverticulitis

Many people go to the doctor and receive a diagnosis of diverticulitis. The diverticulum is nothing more than an abnormally stretched and dilated portion of the bowel that forms a bulging pouch. Most often, it forms in the lower part of the large intestine or descending colon just above the sigmoid flexure. Sometimes there may be more than one diverticulum in various parts of the bowel. Babies are actually born with a diverticulum in the bowels of their body.

Overeating and overfilling the intestinal tract contribute in a way to the development of a diverticulum in the colon. Diverticulitis is characterized by the diverticulum becoming inflamed and beginning to form a sore area or ulcerated areas in the colon. The proper bulk in the colon will help to keep this cleaned out. In many cases, bran will work. In some cases, where the problem is very acute, bran will actually help to plug it up more. In most cases with diverticulitis, a headache is very common, along with fever and bloody stools. It is a problem that develops over the years and needs to be taken care of immediately. Fresh vegetables, vegetables juices, and some fruit will help to correct this problem. Strained green drinks help; chlorophyll is very good, as are cayenne, goldenseal, myrrh, and chaparral.

Colitis

Colitis is an inflammation of the large bowel or intestine, and it may be caused by having too much mucous in the system. It's usually caused by eating the wrong types of foods. Sugars, white flour, and sodas are some of the major offenders. Chocolate is a very serious cause, as are coffee and many other junk foods.

In most cases, operations do help the situation but not the original cause. A person needs to understand the benefits of a proper natural diet and the use of herbs. Most of the people walking around today have a prolapsed colon to some degree; that is a colon that is not staying in the correct position.

Gallbladder and Liver

Cleaning the liver bile ducts is the most powerful procedure that you can do to improve your body's health. But who thinks about that as part of their spring cleaning? ☺

The gallbladder is a small, pear-shaped organ that averages three to six inches in length. It lies underneath the liver in the upper right side of the abdomen. It is connected to the liver and small intestine by small tubes called bile ducts. Bile, a greenish-brown fluid, is utilized by the body to digest fatty foods and assists in the absorption of certain vitamins and minerals. The gallbladder serves as a reservoir for bile. Between meals, bile accumulates and is concentrated within this organ. During meals, the gallbladder contracts and empties bile into the intestine to assist in digestion.

The removal of the gallbladder is a common surgery and those who have had this done need to change their diet and add in enzyme supplements to aid in digestion.

Gallstones

Gallstones are lumps of solid material that form within the gallbladder. There are two major types of gallstones: 1. Cholesterol gallstones are composed mainly of cholesterol, which is made in the liver. These account for nearly 80% of all cases of gallstones in the United States. 2. Pigment gallstones are composed of calcium salts, bilirubin, and other material. They account for the remaining 20% of gallstones in this country.

Here is how gallstones form. Excess cholesterol is removed from the blood by the liver and is then secreted into bile. When bile contains too much cholesterol, small crystals form in bile and they fall to the bottom of the gallbladder. This is like adding too much sugar to coffee and finding sugar at the bottom of the cup. Cholesterol crystals fuse together in the gallbladder to form stones of varying sizes. Pigment gallstones are formed by the secretion of excess bile pigments and bilirubin. The excess pigments and bilirubin form crystals in the gallbladder.

Gallstones vary in size. They may be as small as tiny specks or as large as a small ball. The vast majority measure less than 20 mm, about 1 inch, across. Over time, gallstones may grow in size and/or numbers. However, many gallstones remain the same size for years. Gallbladder sludge occurs when multiple crystals of cholesterol and bilirubin pigments accumulate within the gallbladder but do not fuse together to form a gallstone. Gallbladder sludge typically occurs with fasting and resolves spontaneously. In some, but not all people, gallbladder sludge can develop into gallstones. In the majority of cases, gallbladder sludge is asymptomatic. However, sludge may cause symptoms identical to those attributed to gallstones.

Suggestions

Diet*:

- Increase your intake of vegetables, fruits, and high-fiber foods, especially those containing soluble fiber. Fruits, vegetables, whole grains, legumes, and nuts/seeds are low in saturated fat and high fiber foods that are needed in the diet for healing gallbladder disorders.
- Raw vegetables are good sources of fiber because they contain the cellulose the body needs to break down the fiber. The best source is raw carrots; their fiber binds many colon toxins.
- Red Beets are one of the best foods to support the liver and gallbladder. Carrots are excellent for liver rejuvenation and cleansing.
- Kale can ease liver congestion.
- Apples (especially green) cleanse the liver and gallbladder.
- Blueberries are excellent for the liver and blood.
- Coconut oil can be used by anyone, but it is especially good for those suffering from gallbladder disorders or for anyone who has had their gallbladder removed. Using coconut oil in place of other oils will greatly benefit anyone. Because coconut oil is made of medium chain fatty acids (MCFA), the metabolism of these fatty acids does not require bile or pancreatic enzymes. Therefore, the fats from coconut oil are easily digested with or without a gallbladder.
- A high fiber diet protects from gallbladder disease by binding cholesterol and bile salts and decreasing intestinal transit time. A high fiber diet can only be achieved with unprocessed, unrefined foods.
- Gallbladder disease may be prevented by increased intake of vitamin C and drinking plenty of fresh, "live" juices.

*Unfortunately, the typical American diet provides very little of the needed foods daily.

Suggested supplements:

- Milk thistle, which is a liver detoxifier, helps the liver regenerate and detoxify.
- Lecithin not only maintains the integrity of liver cells but also may help regenerate damaged tissue and normalize bile function.
- Alfalfa is a liver cleanser, rich in vitamins and minerals.

- Fiber binds cholesterol and bile salts.
- Omega is required of every living cell and is needed for repair and prevention of gallstones
- B-complex—All B vitamins are necessary for proper digestion.
- Vitamin C—vitamin C deficiency can lead to gallstones.
- Turmeric helps tone the liver and is known as a liver regenerator.

For those of you who want to make sure your liver is working properly, a liver cleanse might be the answer you want. On the Designed Healthy Living Web site you will find instructions for completing a Liver Cleanse on your own.

FUNCTIONS OF THE LIVER

Toxin terminator – this is what the liver should be known as. It does over 500 different tasks to help you sustain life. Here is a short list of its duties.

Detoxification of:
- Toxic chemicals
- Alcohol
- Allergens
- Microbes
- Microbial antigens
- Drugs
- Hormones
- Antigen-antibody complexes
- Microbial metabolites

Metabolism
Production of:

- Bile
- Cholesterol for sex hormones and adrenal hormones
- Globulin
- Albumin
- Blood-clotting Factors
- Glucose tolerance factor
- Glutathione

Conversion of:

- Glucose to glycogen
- Glycogen to glucose

- Amino acids to glucose
- Fat to energy
- Glucose to fat
- Fat to phospholipids
- Beta-carotene to vitamin A
- Synthesis of nonessential amino acids

Storage & Transports
- Glycogen
- Blood
- Vitamins B12, A, D, E, K. Folate
- Iron, zinc, copper, magnesium

Symptoms of a Sluggish Liver
- Premenstrual syndrome (depression, irritability, mood swings, fatigue, tender breasts, fluid retention, etc.)
- Fibrocystic breasts
- Food allergies
- Chemical hypersensitivities
- Being overweight
- Acne
- Elevated blood cholesterol
- Fatigue
- Depression
- Headache
- Dizziness
- Nausea
- Bad Breath
- Constipation
- Bloating
- Greasy, fatty stools
- Intolerance of fatty foods
- Light or clay-colored stools
- Very dark urine
- Yellowish skin or sclera
- Tender or swollen liver
- Gallbladder problems

- Achy joints and muscles
- Sore feet
- Slow wound healing
- Itching
- Peeling skin
- Dry skin
- Burning feet
- Rashes
- Psoriasis
- Bitter taste in the mouth
- Unexplainable worry or nightmares
- Hypoglycemia
- Bowel toxicity
- Fat-soluble vitamin deficiency (A, D, E, and K)
- Essential fatty acids deficiency

To know how well your liver is functioning, there is a Liver Detoxification Test on the Designed Healthy Living Web site (www.designedhealthyliving.com). This will give you a general idea of the health of your liver. There are specific tests your physician can order to give you a more definitive answer if you have concerns.

Irritable Bowel Syndrome

IBS, Irritable Bowel Syndrome, simply means that the bowel is irritable and not functioning properly. Muscles in the bowel normally contract a few times a day with normal elimination. In a person with IBS, these muscles are extremely sensitive to stimuli or triggers such as food and stress. The person may experience pain, constipation, or diarrhea after eating a salad; whereas, this would not affect a person without IBS. IBS is commonly characterized by abdominal pain and altered bowel function such as constipation, diarrhea, or alternating diarrhea with constipation. IBS is second to the common cold as the most frequent cause of absenteeism from work or school. This disorder can affect people of all ages and backgrounds but is most prevalent in ages 25–45.

Symptoms:

- Abdominal Pain
- Bloating
- Flatulence
- Mucus in the stools
- Anorexia
- Constipation/diarrhea
- Intolerances to certain foods
- Nausea

Possible Contributors to IBS
- Rule out underlying conditions such as Candida, parasites, diverticular disease, infectious diarrhea, lactose intolerance, celiac disease, and infection in small intestine from bacterial overgrowth.
- Food sensitivities and allergies are very common in IBS sufferers. The most common allergens are dairy products and grains—especially wheat and corn. Other possible food triggers are coffee, tea, citrus, and chocolate. Food sensitivity can be discovered by an elimination diet.
- Diet: refined sugar and high fat meals—a rapid rise in blood sugar levels causes a decrease in the intestinal contractions that move food through the GI tract; therefore, there is a type of paralysis in the first two segments of the small intestine, resulting in constipation. Fatty foods may stimulate the colon to empty soon after a meal, before complete digestion has occurred.
- Hormonal Changes—women seem to have more flare-ups around their menstrual cycles.
- Medications—Antibiotics are well known to cause GI problems and diarrhea. They also disturb the balance of intestinal flora in the intestine.
- Low Fiber diets can be a main contributor to IBS. Fiber speeds the transit time of food through the intestinal tract. So food is not sitting in your colon for long periods of time producing toxins and causing more problems.

Inflammatory Bowel Disease (IBD), Crohn's Disease, Ulcerative Colitis

Definition: Diseases that attack the walls of the bowel, causing inflammation. Depending on the location, the disease can be given a number of different names, such as colitis, ulcerative colitis, Crohn's disease, etc. Some specialists call it "arthritis of the intestines."

Symptoms:
- Inflammation
- Open sores
- Bloody, watery stools or hard dry stools
- Diarrhea
- Abdominal pain, bloated, belching, tenderness
- Anemia
- Sharp pains in rectum
- Coated tongue
- Ulcers—followed by a scarred area called stricture (scar tissue)
- Bowel movements come less than sixty minutes after a meal and sometimes during.

(The meal activates the entire intestine.)
- Typically IBD is divided into two main categories:
    - Crohn's disease—involves the layers of tissues in the bowel and affects the entire GI tract – it is related to a refined diet with high sugar and corn allergy
    - Ulcerative Colitis—affects the colon or rectum only

Possible Causes:
- Serious bout with flu or some other virus or illness
- Emotional involvement and stress. Both cause hormonal changes. A hormonal imbalance then causes changes in immune system. There is a strong correlation between stress and flare-ups.
- Deficiency of EPA (Omega-3). Under these conditions the immune system makes a mistake and starts to attack the body's own tissues. This can result in arthritis, psoriasis, or IBD. People whose diets are rich in EPA don't get IBD. EPA comes mainly from cold-water fish, such as mackerel, haddock, sardines, salmon, and tuna. Flax seed ground daily also gives a great amount of Omega-3.
- Toxic Chemicals
- Malfunctioning immune system

Special Concerns:
- Mal-absorption of nutrients, especially B-complex, iron, zinc, and calcium
- Fear of flare ups if one chooses to eat poorly
- Fiber Matrix: There is a tough resistant part of certain foods that is so tough it passes through one's intestine without being broken down (digested). This fiber matrix can irritate an inflamed and sensitive intestine tremendously. Examples of this are corn, berries with seeds, unpeeled apples or pears, nuts, crisp veggies, grapes, potato skins, etc.
- Strictures and blockages—places of inflammation can heal; however, scar tissue develops on the intestine. This scar tissue can cause the fiber matrix to stop or pull at this place. This hurts! One can have diarrhea or constipation.
- Medication—has side effects and causes nutrient deficiencies
- People with IBD are usually lactose intolerant (inability to digest milk and sugar), so they avoid milk and dairy products. Yogurt is usually all right for them.

Chemicals that Trigger IBD

- Additives in carbonated beverages (the preservative benzoic acid)
- Medicines—antibiotics, non-steroidal anti-inflammatory, BCP, gold, sulphasalazine
- Fluoride
- Environmental pollution
- Preservatives and food additives
- Synthetic chemicals
- Toxic metals, such as aluminum and mercury and plastics
- Vaccinations

Nutritional Guidelines for Healing

It is best to read about each source of nutrition in the Nutrition and Vitamin sections of this manual.

- EPA—anti-inflammatory, reduces inflammation, anti-fungal,
- Peppermint – best remedy for stomach, increase bile and stomach lining
- Calcium—helps stop diarrhea
- Diet – eat lots of vegetables, avocados, sweet potatoes and apples
- Water – proper amount of filtered water.
- Protein—eggs, chicken, fish, yogurt, soy protein drink
- Zinc—Vital nutrient for building one's immune system, production of one's digestive enzymes, and hormones
- Good multivitamin—with at least 12 vitamins and 7 minerals
- Folic Acid—Take in a B-Complex or whole food source. Drugs used to control intestinal flare-ups interfere with folic acid absorption. This increases the risk of cancer by 50%.
- Fiber—essential in supplemental form unless grinding and making your own bread
- Vitamin E—always deficient in those with IBD. Will help dissolve scar tissue.
- Vitamin C—Most with IBD are avoiding fruits because of fiber problems. Take a sustained vitamin C.
- Natural anti-inflammatory – to reduce swelling and inflammation

CANDIDA

Many alternative and preventative health care practitioners find that a surprisingly high number of chronic health concerns are related to an overgrowth of yeast in the body (Candida albicans). To see if you have this underlying problem, read the information here and then go to the Designed Healthy Living Web site to take the Candida Test (under the Happy and Healthy tab).

Cause

This overgrowth occurs when we disturb the natural balance in the body:

- By introducing antibiotics; hormones, including birth control pills; steroid-based medications, i.e. cortisone; or chemotherapy.
- By consuming diets high in sugars and refined carbohydrates and/or too low in fresh fruits and vegetables (3–5 servings a day recommended), fad diets, or stress.

Result—Yeast Overgrowth

The result is yeast, which normally coexists with friendly bacteria (lactobacillus and bifidus) in the gut and other mucosal membranes of the body, grows out of control. The yeast feeds on the sugars and carbohydrates, while the friendly, but fragile, bacteria that normally keep the yeast in check are easily destroyed by medications, intestinal disturbances, stress, etc.

Listed below are the symptoms that may mean Candida is a concern for you to consider. As I mentioned, there is a Candida questionnaire and score sheet located on the Designed Healthy Living Web site, www.designedhealthyliving.com. I encourage you to take this test and have each member of your family take it also. The intense research of William Crook, M.D. helped develop this questionnaire to more accurately identify whether or not someone is dealing with Candida. After knowing your score, the suggestions listed below to get back in balance are a great starting point. You may find it helpful to work with a medical professional to get full control of this health interference.

Symptoms—Brain/Nervous System:

- Anxiety
- Headaches
- Mood swings
- Poor mental focus
- Depression
- Irritability
- Poor memory
- Dizziness

Symptoms—Digestive:

- Colitis/irritable bowel disease
- Constipation

- Belching
- Bloating/ gas
- Bad breath

- Diarrhea
- Abdominal pain

Symptoms—Immune/ Respiratory:

- Frequent infection, especially ears/tonsils
- Sinus congestion
- Pain/tightness in chest
- Asthma-like symptoms
- Mucous in stools
- Cravings for sweets, breads
- Redness around rectal area

- Chronic cough
- Environmental sensitivities, i.e. mold
- Heartburn
- Rectal itching
- Food allergies

Symptoms—Reproductive:

- Endometriosis
- Cervical dysplasia
- Infertility
- Prostatitis
- Pelvic pain

- Uterine fibroids
- PMS
- Loss of libido
- Impotence
- Vaginal discharge/itching

Other Symptoms:

- Acne/ skin disorders
- Athlete's foot
- Canker sores
- Rash/blisters in mouth
- Joint pain/arthritis
- Diabetes
- Spots in front of eyes

- White coated tongue
- Nail fungus
- Burning tongue
- Fatigue
- Muscle aches/ weakness
- Blurred vision

Getting Back in Balance

- Reduce yeast growth by increasing friendly bacteria (yogurt).
- Increase your garlic consumption.
- Take a pre and probiotic supplement (must state: "active cultures at time of absorption in intestine").
- Take B-complex.
- Strengthen the immune system with a good quality vitamin/mineral supplement.

"Die Off"

Be aware that when the yeast "dies off," toxins are released that can cause headaches, fatigue, achy joints, diarrhea, or any of the other yeast overgrowth symptoms. Make sure you are getting plenty of fiber in your diet to increase bowel movements to quickly move the toxins out of your body.

Candida Diet

1. *Remove foods that feed yeast*: sugars—maple syrup, honey, molasses, and corn syrup—and refined carbohydrates—white flour products, including crackers, snacks, and chips.

2. *Include foods that nourish cells*: protein-rich foods—poultry (free range, lean and not ground), fish (wild), and eggs (free range and fresh).

3. *Eat Low-Carb vegetables*: look for fresh and without mold—dark salad greens, spinach, asparagus, avocados, broccoli, cauliflower, green beans, Brussels sprouts, peppers, summer squash, and cucumbers.

4. *Pass up the fruits.*

5. *Adjust your condiments*: select olive oil, spices, herbs, and sea salt. Good spices and herbs to choose are basil, cumin, garlic, ginger root, horseradish, onion, and oregano.

6. *Stock up on some frozen vegetables* such as frozen artichoke hearts or green peas. Use them for soups and salads. Check labels, and avoid those with sugar, vinegar, and additives.

7. *Deli*: Select corn tortillas and shun everything else. Avoid preservatives.

8. *Crackers*: look for yeast and sugar free whole grain crackers, typically found in the health food store.

9. *Seeds, nuts, legumes, and grains*: be sure to use brown rice and whole grains.

DIABETES

Diabetes is an Epidemic in North America

Did you know?

- Diabetes kills approximately 350,000 North Americans per year.
- It is the third largest killer after heart disease and cancer.

- Diabetes is the number one cause of blindness in North America.
- Vitamin D in pregnancy and in young children prevents diabetes.

Two Types of Diabetes:

Type 1—Juvenile diabetes, representing 10% of diagnosed cases. Known causes include:

- damaged beta cells in pancreas caused by viral infections (flu, mumps, chicken pox, measles).
- environmental chemicals.
- stress.
- genetic issues (it's inherited).

Type 2—once called "Adult Onset," but now it is affecting our children, representing 90% of diagnosed cases. This type of diabetes is totally diet related and preventable.

There are two types of type 2 diabetes:

- Insulin* Dependent—caused by not enough insulin being manufactured by the pancreas.
- Insulin Resistant—caused by insulin receptors malfunctioning, or insulin receptors missing.

To reduce the risk of developing type 2 diabetes, we must maintain a good blood sugar level, which is dependent on four things:

- A wise diet—including adequate fiber and avoidance of simple carbohydrates.
- A healthy pancreas.
- Healthy adrenal glands.
- Exercise.

The pancreas makes insulin. Insulin is the "door-man" for the cell—it opens the door and allows glucose into the cell. In order to have a healthy pancreas, it is essential to consume adequate nutrients, especially protein, vitamin C, B vitamins, and zinc.

The "Insulin Receptor Sites" on the cell can be compared to "door-knobs." Insulin resistant diabetics often have:

- "Missing door-knobs." This is usually due to lack of nutrients (minerals, B vitamins, and all of the amino acids) and a dirty liver. Therefore, alfalfa, B-complex, soy protein, and herbs such as milk thistle are recommended.
- "Door-knobs" covered with fat. Therefore, they are malfunctioning, and insulin cannot open the door to allow glucose in. Weight loss is essential to assist this situation.

Diabetics take warning: Insulin does not cure diabetes, it keeps you alive. This means you need to be proactive in regards to your diet and exercise to maintain a healthy life.

Due to more understanding of blood sugar, diabetics rarely die from elevated blood sugar levels now as they did in the past. However, instead, they have to contend with the long-term complications of the disease that will happen in five to fifteen years unless steps are taken to prevent or reduce the complications.

Complications of Diabetes:

1. *Heart Disease*—narrowing of large arteries that supply the heart + increased risk of strokes + high cholesterol and triglycerides due to high sugar level in blood

2. *Peripheral Vascular Disease*—poor circulation to the legs and feet, leading to gangrene and amputations

3. *Retinopathy*—narrowing and breakage of blood vessels in the eyes, leading to blindness

4. *Neuropathy*—tingling, burning, numbness, and pins and needles sensations, especially in legs and feet

5. *Kidney Problems*—due to high sugar in urine. Kidney failure is the cause of death for many diabetics.

6. *High Blood Pressure*—due to narrowing of the blood vessels

7. *Infections*—diabetics are more prone to infections and often don't heal well.

Reduce or Prevent the Impact of Diabetes on your life!

- Exercise removes glucose from the blood without insulin.
- Follow the Healthy Treasures Fresh Market Pyramid with a limited amount of sugar.
- Take supplements to reduce or prevent the complications, as well as help prevent disease.
- Since obesity can affect insulin receptor sites, get weight under control.
- Don't smoke! It causes constriction of the arteries.
- Eliminate sugar from the diet.

Suggested Supplements:

1. *Soy Protein*—low fat protein source, essential for healthy insulin receptor sites

2. *Multiple Vitamin*—vitamin and mineral smorgasbord

3. *Fiber* slows down glucose absorption into blood.

4. *Omega, Lecithin, and Milled Flaxseed* are helpful for neuropathy symptoms and reduce heart disease risk.

5. *Vitamin E* improves circulation, helps reduce risk of clotting, reduces risk of retinopathy and neuropathy, and reduces oxidation—thereby, reducing LDL cholesterol.

6. *B Complex*-reduces neuropathy reduces plaque formation in arteries, increases glucose utilization, and increases immunity.

7. *Vitamin C* is a natural infection fighter, improves healing, and is essential for health of the eyes and kidneys.

8. *Alfalfa* is an excellent source of minerals. Diabetics experience excess mineral loss due to frequent urination.

9. *Zinc* is essential for pancreas health and to increase the body's immune function.

10. *Beta Carotene* is good for the eyes.

Complications will happen with *all* diabetics (usually within five to fifteen years), unless they do something to prevent them. *It is worth the investment in quality of life to make the necessary changes!*

HEART HEALTH

For it is with your heart that you believe and are justified, and it is with your mouth that you confess and are saved.

Romans 10:10 NIV

Heart Facts

DO YOU LOVE your heart? Weighing in at 10 ounces, the blood-filled muscle called the heart has become the universal symbol of love.

Do you love to laugh? Have you ever had the kind of laugh that sends a stream of tears from your eyes? It warms our soul and has great benefits, too. Research has shown that a good "belly laugh" can cause the lining of blood vessel walls called endothelium to relax; increasing blood flow for up to forty-five minutes after the laugh attack. Damage to the endothelium can lead to the narrowing of blood vessels and eventually cardiovascular diseases. That's no laughing matter…or maybe it is.

Do you love power? In under a minute, your heart can pump blood to every cell in your body. And over the course of a day, about 100,000 heart beats shuttle 2,000 gallons of oxygen-rich blood many times through about 60,000 miles of branching blood vessels that link together the cells of our organs and body parts. That's a hefty job for a fist-sized muscle.

Do you have a broken heart? A broken heart can cause one to swoon. A breakup with a loved one or news of a family member's death literally can lead to broken hearts in the form of heightened risk for heart attack, studies have shown. Such trauma can also trigger the release of stress hormones into the bloodstream that temporarily "stun" the heart. The resulting symptoms mimic those of a heart attack—chest pain and shortness of breath—but this type of achy heart can bounce back in days with some TLC and rest.

Do you want to protect your heart? In this reading you will learn the about the two most prevalent problems that lead to heart problems: cardiovascular disease and elevated cholesterol. If you love your heart, then you will want to follow the advice given for a healthy diet and exercise program.

Cardiovascular Disease

Definition:

1. Arteriosclerosis, or Hardening of the Arteries
2. Hypertension or High Blood Pressure
3. Rheumatic Heart Disease

Cardiovascular disease is the #1 cause of death in the United States. Cancer is a close second.

Begins with:

Insult or injury in the inner layer of an artery. This insult or injury can be due to:

- toxins
- viral infections
- trauma or stress
- chemicals
- radiation

Do you notice that these factors may happen without your even being aware of them? This means that the heart injury or insult can happen to anyone regardless of age, race, health, etc. These are all factors that do not include diet. The diet will play a big role from this point forward in heart disease.

Our bodies respond:

Our body begins laying down cholesterol or a plaque to heal this insult. This thickens and narrows the opening of arteries, resulting in high blood pressure or high cholesterol.

Notes:

- Calcium/Magnesium reduces high blood pressure.
- Vitamin E/Selenium increases oxygen to the heart muscle, decreases the clot, and may prevent this from happening in the first place.
- Vitamin C increases elasticity in muscles, including the heart.

Results:

Turbulence begins and the flow of blood slows. Cells (platelets) clump together forming a clot, blocking the vessels. If the coronary artery is blocked, a heart attack occurs. If the cerebral (brain) artery is blocked, a stroke occurs. *Ninety percent of heart attacks are caused by clots.*

Additional Contributions to Heart Disease

1. Improper Diet:

    Trans fats, hydrogenated, partially hydrogenated oils, heated oils

    Processed meat—preservatives, nitrates, nitrites

    Medicated meats—animals loaded with chemicals in feed and living in concentration camps

    Fried foods

    Processed dairy foods—homogenized milk is the main contributor to the plaque

    Refined white sugar

    Excessive salt

    Alcohol

    Not enough fruits, veggies, nuts, seeds, whole grains

2. Smoking: Do not smoke. People who smoke are 2–3 times more likely to have a heart attack.

3. Stress: See information in this book to learn more about stress.

4. Related or other health concerns.

5. Lack of exercise

6. Being overweight

7. High homocysteine levels

Rebuilding your health or reversing cardiovascular disease

1. Tiny amounts of aspirin inhibit the clumping of platelets. However, taking aspirin increases the number of hemorrhagic strokes (bleeding into the brain). Fruits and veggies have just the right amount of aspirin to prevent both kinds of strokes. Just three raw veggies* a day, one cup serving each, decreases the incidence of strokes and heart attacks by a significant amount.

* Certain foods are wonderful at inhibiting platelet clumping. These include fresh onions, garlic, wild fish, and pineapple.

2. Stay at normal weight

3. Exercise

4. Eat natural fats not processed fats. Butter vs. margarine, etc.

5. Eat more soluble fiber. Soluble fibers bind cholesterol-rich bile acids and cause them to be excreted from the body when they would otherwise be reabsorbed.

6. Give your body adequate amounts of proper nutrients.

Supplement Guide for a Healthy Heart:

- Calcium, Magnesium
- Co Q 10
- EPA
- Fiber
- Lecithin
- Soy Protein
- Vitamin C
- Vitamin E

Lipids

Lipids are fat-like substances found in the body's cells and in the bloodstream. Often referred to as cholesterol and triglycerides, lipids are an important source of fuel for the body. They contain dietary fatty acids, cholesterol, vitamins A, D, E and K, and choline, lecithin, Co-Q-10, phospholipids and more.

If your diet is healthy, your lipids (lipoproteins) are full of essential fats, vitamins and all kinds of really good stuff. But if you eat bad fats - processed oils - your lipids will carry these bad fats around your body so the cholesterol numbers get out of whack. This causes HDL to go down and LDL and triglycerides to go up. As you may already know, there are several ways your doctor can measure your lipid levels to understand your risk of developing heart disease. Through a standard blood test, your doctor can check:

- Triglycerides: Triglycerides are stored in your body fat and come from the fats and oils that you eat. High triglycerides are usually associated with high sugar and together they contribute to inflammation and disease. Normal triglycerides are considered less than 150 mg/dL.
- HDL, "Good" cholesterol: HDL is known as the good cholesterol because it helps sweep "bad" cholesterol out of the body. The higher your HDL, the better. HDL should be above 45 mg/dL in men, and above 50mg/dL in women.

- LDL, "Bad" cholesterol: LDL is known as the bad cholesterol, because high LDL leads to clogged arteries and heart disease. Optimal levels of LDL are less than three times the HDL level. For example: HDL 50 then the LDL should be less than 150.
- Total cholesterol is not as important as the individual numbers themselves. Refer to the HDL, LDL and triglycerides before considering a cellular altering drug. Changing to a diet free of altered fats - fats that are not in the natural state - will drastically change these numbers more so than the drugs.

Another way to decipher cholesterol numbers is through a fairly new study just reaching the American doctor offices: APOB (apolipoprotein B) blood test and non-HDL cholesterol (total cholesterol minus HDL cholesterol).

Non-HDL, "Total bad" cholesterol:

Non-HDL is the measure of all the lipids in your blood, except HDL, the "good" cholesterol. It measures the level of *all* the "bad" cholesterol combined. Normal non-HDL-C levels should be 30 mg/dL above LDL. In other words, if your target LDL is 100 mg/dL, your target non-HDL-C would be 130 mg/dL. If the total is 200 minus 60 (HDL) = 140 non-HDL. This means the total needs to be lowered through diet, exercise, and supplementation, and the HDL needs to be raised to bring the non-HDL to a number lower then 130.

An Assignment for You

It is imperative to realize that you are in charge of your health. The best way to track progress is to keep a record of blood profiles and make notes of changes made in your diet, exercise, and supplementation. Your physician cannot be your chef, personal trainer, and psychologists all in one. *You* will need to take charge of *your* health. Keeping a record of your results for years will help you and your physician determine when the proper use of drug treatment is necessary and when you can make changes to avoid the treatment.

Lowering Cholesterol Naturally

Dietary Changes

Fresh Fruits and vegetables
- Raw or lightly steamed

Whole grains
- Brown rice
- Organically grown, no white stuff!

Soy - organic
- High-quality, minimally processed

Change your fats
- Eat natural fats: organic butter, essential oils, olive oil, clean fish, etc.
- Increase the good fats.
- Omega-3 fatty acids (sardines, anchovies, etc.)
- Olive oil (extra virgin—cold pressed)

Lifestyle Changes
- Stop smoking. Smoking increases oxidation of cholesterol, which is not good.
- Exercise: exercises increases HDL in cholesterol, which is good.
- Maintain **ideal weight**: Obese adults have 50–100 % increased risk of premature death. Even moderate weight reductions (5–10%) lower the risk of death from all heart diseases. Abdominal obesity (over 40 inches in men, over 35 inches in women) is a great contributor to heart disease and diabetes.
- Cravings for sweets and refined carbohydrates are sometimes not related to will-power but to metabolic imbalances. Read more about insulin resistance under Diabetes in this manual.

Fiber
Fiber, especially soluble fibers, bind with cholesterol—rich bile acids, preventing them from being absorbed into the blood, thus lowering blood cholesterol levels naturally

Supplements Can Help
Omega-3
- Helps reduce 3 major risk factors:
  - elevated blood pressure
  - elevated triglycerides
  - elevated cholesterol
- Reduces inflammation in coronary arteries
  - first step in plaque formation
  - measured by C-reactive protein

Make sure the supplement you choose is:

- Readily absorbed (bioavalable).
- Clinically tested (that means on people not animals before marketing).
- Odor controlled.
- Free from heavy metals.
- One with an excellent proportion of EPA (545 mg) and DHA (235mg) plus additional Omega-3 fatty acids.
- Easy to digest.

Garlic

- helps lower cholesterol and triglycerides
- raises HDL
- is an anti-inflammatory
- increases blood fluidity

A good garlic supplement:
- Releases allicin (active ingredient) past the stomach, so as to avoid being destroyed by stomach acids
- Uses a cool-dried process which retains all the potency of raw garlic without odor

Soy Protein

- Isoflavones in soy reduce cholesterol.
- Look for a soy protein that uses water washed soy, thus retaining high levels of isoflavones.
- An excellent protein alternative
- Contains only non-GMO—soy tightly monitored and controlled from planting to harvesting
- Protect LDL from oxidizing

Pro-Biotic

- Contains acidophilus and bifidus, essential bacteria for the intestines
- Helps prevent reabsorption of cholesterol from the lower intestines
- Triple encapsulated to protect from stomach acids, oxygen, and moisture
- High levels of micro flora help improve HDL/LDL ratio.

The bottle *must* state "guaranteed live bacteria delivered to the intestine tract."

Cholesterol Lowering Drugs

Possible side effects of statin drugs:

- Back pain
- Constipation
- Dizziness
- Hair loss
- Impotence
- Insomnia
- Liver damage
- Muscle damage, pain
- Sore throat
- Tiredness
- Blurred vision
- Diarrhea
- Dry eyes
- Headaches
- Indigestion, heartburn
- Kidney damage
- Muscle cramps
- Nerve damage
- Stomach pain, nausea
- Weakness

Heart Healthy Nutrients

B-Complex*

B-complex helps reduce homocysteine in the blood stream, which may be a greater contributor to heart disease than even cholesterol. High homocysteine levels can significantly increase risk for:

- Strokes in large vessels.
- Small strokes in the brain that result in mental deficiency.
- Direct damage in lining blood vessels reducing blood flow to the brain.
- Blockage in deep veins (thrombosis).
- Blockages in arteries of arms, hands, legs, and feet.
- 50% increase in risk of heart attack.

Carotenoids *
CoQ-10 *—prevent LDL oxidation (60% of Americans are deficient)
Vitamin E *

* These supplements are explained in this manual in "Value Your Vitamins."

Make a commitment to your health today—be your healthiest you!

IMMUNE SYSTEM

O UR BODIES CONTINUALLY strive to maintain optimal health. It has an internal wisdom that knows what to do in case of injury or an invasion of any bad guys (viruses, bacteria, parasites, etc.). As long as these injuries or invasions are not too overwhelming, the body does just fine fending for itself. It knows how to make its own bandages, called scabs. It knows how to make its own warriors, called antibodies, to fight injury. Obviously, at times the body needs some help to accomplish its mission of healing, but even after the stitches, it's the body's internal mechanisms that eventually heal the wound. It's the body that eventually deals with the invading bacteria with the antibodies and brings itself back to health. The trick to all this miraculous healing ability of the body is to have a strong, healthy, optimal-functioning immune system.

Factors that weaken the immune system:
- Antibiotic use
- Candida
- Chronic infections or allergies
- Lack of nutrients such as high-quality protein, water, and vitamins
- Obesity
- Ongoing stress
- Pollutants or toxins in food and environment
- Poor digestion or absorption
- Saturated – trans fats
- Skin disorders such as eczema
- Smoking
- Sugar

Ways to support your immune system:
- Optimal amounts of essential nutrients like vitamins A, B, C, D, and E
- Increase antioxidant intake—C and E.
- Maintain a healthy balance of intestinal microflora—probiotics, yogurt.
- Eat garlic—great immune system support.
- Exercise.
- Vitamin D
- Zinc
- Maintain acid balance on your skin—pH balanced body products.
- Investigate underlying issues such as allergies, Candida, and chronic problems.

Trouble with Tonsils

Many of us have been led to believe that the tonsils are not a vital organ and that if they become infected "one too many times," they should be removed. Well, your immune system begs to differ. Tonsils are a vital part of your immune system. They are small masses of lymphatic tissue found in the mucous lining around the throat. Their job is to trap and remove bacteria and/or pathogens that enter via the throat. They are so good at their job that occasionally they become congested with bad guys, in which case they become red, swollen, and painful. If this occurs, your body is letting you know you have an immune battle on your hands. This is the time for you to provide optimal support and include rest, high levels of nutrients, probiotics, garlic, and fluids. It is also time to review your lifestyle to decide if you are "overtaxing" your immune system. If you remove your first line of defense to your respiratory tract, you have removed your front line army and put more responsibility and pressure on the other troops.[53]

ALLERGIES AND SINUS RELIEF PROGRAM

Most people who suffer with allergy and sinus problems feel that they must resort to using medications that have unpleasant and even dangerous side effects. For those who are interested in safer, more natural alternatives, some of the following natural solutions may help.

Each of these vitamins and herbs has more information in this book. As you continue to learn about these natural solutions, you will discover the foods highest in each nutrient.

Garlic
- Natural antibiotic
- normalizes and stabilizes the immune system
- encourages normal mucous production

Vitamin C
- Natural antihistamine and a histamine stabilizer
- Reduces mucous and congestion
- Anti-inflammatory, helps prevent narrowing of bronchial tubes
- Enhances T-cell and macrophage function
- Is a mast cell wall stabilizer
- Improves tissue oxygenation and promotes healing

Natural Interferon
- Supports and stimulates the immune system be increasing the activity of macrophages (white blood cells) and inducing natural inferno production. It optimizes the body's immune response against environmental irritants and airborne substances.
- Completely safe, no adverse reactions to these plant extracts
- Natural plant extracts derived from pumpkin seeds, safflower flowers, plantago seeds, Japanese honeysuckle flower buds

Alfalfa
- Source of fiber that helps in binding toxins and carrying out of body
- Natural chlorophyll
- Natural antihistamine
- Decongestant
- Anti-inflammatory
- Natural diuretic

Probiotic
- Enhances the body's total immune response
- Reduce the consumption of dairy products, since they tend to increase mucous production.

Reduce Exposure to Toxins
- Purify the air in your home and office with an Air Purifier.
- Use organic, safe cleaners in your home, laundry, and dishes.
- Use natural, pH-balanced skin care products.

For allergy and sinus relief in the winter, when it's dry, remember to use a humidifier with a few drops of Basic G to inhibit bacterial growth.

> Because the brain is the most sensitive organ in the body, many experts recommend eliminating foods and environmental irritants that could create brain allergies."
> –Dr. Doris Rapp, *Is This Your Child's World?*

ADRENAL

Have you ever felt stressed and wondered why? Or have you ever wondered why you cannot lose weight? The answer may lie in the adrenal glands. These glands rest right above the kidneys. They are responsible for regulating stress, metabolism, and blood sugar. Adrenaline is known as the "fight or flight" response. It is responsible for protecting our bodies when in danger or under stress, causing the heart rate to be increased, glucose to be released from its energy stores, and increasing blood flow. When the body is in a constant state of stress, the excess cortisol stimulates glucose production. That excess glucose is then stored as fat, particularly in the abdominal region. Several hormones are released from these glands:

- *Adrenaline (epinephrine)*: helps the body cope with danger and speeds up the rate of metabolism. It gives energy and alertness and is one of the main hormones released in stressful situations.
- *Cortisol*: is involved in the metabolism of carbohydrates and the regulation of blood sugar. It helps produce glucose from proteins and increases energy in times of stress. And it has anti-inflammatory actions.
- *Dehydroepiandrosterone (DHEA)*: is also called an androgen, meaning it can be converted into testosterone; therefore, making it a multi-functioning steroid.
- *Nonepinephrine*: affects the part of the brain where responding and attention actions are controlled.
- *Cortisone*: is a steroid, and can also suppress the immune system.
- *Aldosterone*: helps to maintain electrolyte (salt) imbalances in the body, also secretes potassium.
- *Androstenedione*: helps make estrogen, also an androgen that can be converted into testosterone (steroid).

When the adrenals malfunction, it's referred to as *low adrenal reserve* or adrenal fatigue. Since each person handles stress differently, it is important to understand what lifestyle factors can lead to adrenal fatigue.

Lifestyle Factors contributing to Adrenal Fatigue:[53]
- Lack of sleep
- Processed food diet
- Using food and drinks as stimulants when tired
- Staying up late even though fatigued
- Being constantly in a position of powerlessness
- Constantly driving yourself
- Trying to be perfect
- Staying in no-win situations over time
- Lack of enjoyable and rejuvenating activities

Symptoms of Adrenal Fatigue:[54]
- Difficulty getting up in the morning
- Continuous fatigue not relieved by sleep
- Craving for salt or salty foods
- Lack of energy
- Increased effort to do everyday tasks
- Decreased sex drive
- Decreased ability to handle stress
- Increased time to recover from illness, injury, or trauma
- Light-headed when standing up quickly
- Mild depression
- Less enjoyment or happiness with life
- Increased PMS
- Symptoms increase if meals are skipped or inadequate
- Thoughts less focused, more-fuzzy
- Memory less accurate

Now for the good news, you can do most of what is necessary to recover and regain your adrenal health by yourself. There are no magic pills for this, but there are certainly key lifestyle changes and nutritional supplements that will greatly impact your recovery.

- *Lifestyle*—what you eat, drink, thoughts you feed your mind, and beliefs you base your life on. For this we suggest you study the *Treasures of Healthy Living Bible Study.* This will guide you in understanding how these areas work together and God's specific plan for you.
- *Supplements*—vitamin C (has an enhancing effect on adrenals), vitamin E,

B-Complex, calcium, magnesium, a good foodlet multi vitamin (in other words, a vitamin proven to be from food—not synthetic), fiber, licorice root, ashwagandha root, Panax Ginseng, L-Theanine, and a resveratrol-ellagic blend tonic.

CANCER PREVENTION

Cancer occurs when our bodies are exposed to a factor or combination of factors that damage normal cells and makes them start dividing uncontrollably. In America, it has escalated to epidemic proportions. Below you will see a list of cancer-causing substances, commonly called carcinogens. This is a very short list compared to the actual list of known carcinogens sold in our market.

Items to eliminate or severely limit in your diet*:
- Red Meat: limit to once a week—look for organic without the use of hormones and antibiotics
- Processed meat of any kind—nitrates, hot dogs, luncheon, smoked, or cured meat
- Organ meats—liver, kidney, brains, and such
- Skin of fowl—even clean fowl stores its toxins in the skin and fat layer
- Fried foods
- High-fat dairy products
- Alcohol
- Refined sugar and flour
- Hydrogenated oils

*External and lifestyle factors account for 80% of cancer deaths.

Chemicals to limit exposure to:
- Synthetic estrogens
- Pesticides and herbicides
- Flame retardant clothing
- Artificial preservatives—nitrates, nitrates, nitrosamines
- Solvents
- Chemicals in household products—including disinfectants
- Avoid prescription and OTC—many are minor carcinogenic agents
- Detergents
- Plastics
- Cigarette smoking increases pancreatic cancer

Suggested Food Plan: Be very selective of the foods you choose:

- Fowl with skin removed--free range, farm raised
- Deep sea cold water fish at least three times a week—wild, never farm raised
- Yogurt products—no hormones, antibiotics
- Whole grains—variety of grains per week
- Purified water
- Organic cheese
- Nuts, brown rice
- Cruciferous vegetables—50% of you daily diet is optimal
- Onions, garlic, leeks

Cooking utensils:

- Use only glass for storage.
- Use wooden or stainless steel cooking utensils.
- Use waterless stainless steel cookware or stainless steel—see resource for a supplier.
- Avoid non-stick and aluminum products.
- Avoid the microwave— microwaved foods lead to lower white blood cells which lead to weakened immune system and also lead to anemia.

Supplementing your diet

These supplements are vital to preventing and reducing the cancer cells in your body:

- Vitamins A, C, E; selenium; B-complex; Magnesium; Omega-3; Zinc
- Folic acid reduces breast cancer by 50%
- Soluble fiber
- Beta-carotene
- Natural interferon
- Resveratrol, ellagic acid blend tonic

When diagnosed with cancer, the need for supplements and a diet high in fruits, veggies, and whole grains increases tremendously.

Recommendation and Consultations:

Through nutrition, supplements, and personal coaching, Dr. Sandra Bevacqua guides individuals to obtain and maintain optimal health. She has a Ph.D. in molecular and cellular Biology and has completed many studies at the universities for cancer research. Dr. Bevacqua does consultations for people who wish to use natural products to help them with rebuilding during and after chemo and radiation. She will work with your physician to develop the best nutrition and supplementation program to not counteract the treatment your physician may deem necessary. Her website is www.wish4life.com . This would be my first stop if I was diagnosed with cancer. She has seen some great results.

How cancer cells are fed:

1. Sugar is a cancer-feeder. By cutting off sugar, it cuts off one important food supply to the cancer cells. Sugar substitutes like NutraSweet, Equal, Spoonful, etc. are made with aspartame and may be harmful. A better natural substitute would be Manuka honey, Xagave, or molasses, but only in very small amounts.

2. Milk, homogenized and pasteurized, causes the body to produce mucus, especially in the gastrointestinal tract. Cancer feeds on mucus. Raw milk is a better option since it provides enzymes and essential nutrients.

3. Cancer cells thrive in an acid environment. A meat-based diet is acidic, and it is best to eat fish and a little chicken rather than beef or pork. Meat also contains livestock antibiotics, growth hormones, and parasites, which are all harmful, especially to people with cancer.

4. A diet made of 80% fresh vegetables, especially cruciferous vegetables and juice, whole grains, seeds, nuts, and a little fruit help put the body into an alkaline environment. About 20% can be from cooked food, including beans. Fresh vegetable juices provide live enzymes that are easily absorbed and reach down to cellular levels within fifteen minutes to nourish and enhance growth of healthy cells. To obtain live enzymes for building healthy cells, drink fresh vegetable juice (most vegetables, including bean sprouts), and eat some raw vegetables two or three times a day. Enzymes are destroyed at temperatures of 104 degrees F (40 degrees C).

5. Avoid coffee, tea, and chocolate, which have high caffeine. Green tea is a better alternative and has cancer-fighting properties. Water is best to drink. Drink purified water, or filtered, to avoid known toxins and heavy metals in tap water.

6. Meat protein is difficult to digest and requires a lot of digestive enzymes. Undigested meat remaining in the intestines becomes putrefied and leads to more toxic build-up. Organic pastured meat is still a healthy option.

7. Cancer cell walls have a tough protein covering. By refraining from or eating less medicated meat, it frees more enzymes to attack the protein walls of cancer cells and allows the body's killer cells to destroy the cancer cells.

8. Some supplements build up the immune system (anti-oxidants, vitamins, minerals, EFAs, etc.) to enable the body's own killer cells to destroy cancer cells. Other supplements like vitamin E are known to cause apoptosis, or programmed cell death, the body's normal method of disposing of damaged, unwanted, or unneeded cells.

9. Cancer is a disease of the mind, body, and spirit. A proactive and positive spirit will help the cancer warrior be a survivor. Anger, resentment, and bitterness put the body into a stressful and acidic environment. Learn to have a loving and forgiving spirit. Learn to relax and enjoy life.

10. Cancer cells cannot thrive in an oxygenated environment. Exercising daily and deep breathing promote oxygen delivery to the cellular level. Oxygen therapy is another means employed to destroy cancer cells.

THE CONTROL OF INFLAMMATION

In America, we have a problem, and that problem is an alarming increase of inflammatory diseases that are besieging every age segment of our population. Our children, teenagers, medium adults, and especially our senior adults are experiencing the painful health consequences that these diseases are imposing on them.

For example, more Americans are going to the doctor now than at any other time in our history. We now lead the world in doctor visits. This indicates that we are the sickest country in the world. Let's examine why.

What are inflammatory diseases?

Inflammatory diseases can be defined as any disease that causes an inflammatory response from the immune system. The immune system protects each cell from any foreign or harmful toxin that might enter into your body. The protection afforded by the immune system is amazing. When I lecture to my pre-medical students at Baylor University, I feel unworthy as I ponder the complexity of the system, for it is so awe-inspiring. The immune system is the most complicated, most synchronized, most balanced, and most orderly in its sequence design of any system in the human body. After I finish my lecture, the wonder and amazement on my students' faces is priceless.

Most prevalent Inflammatory Diseases in America

Known		Suspected	Thought	
Arthritis	Colitis	Diabetes	Bronchitis	Alzheimer's
Allergies	Crohn's	Nephritis	Emphysema	Cancer
Asthma	Celiac	Hepatitis		
Dermatitis	Psoriasis	Thyroiditis		
Gout	Atherosclerosis	Osteoarthritis		

As you look over this list, it is likely that you will recognize a disease that you or one of your family members have or have had. As you can see, America definitely has a problem.

What is inflammation?

First, let's begin by looking at the relationship between omega-3 and omega-6 fatty acids. When we eat foods that contain fats, our digestive enzymes breaks the fat down into fatty acids for our cells to use. Two of these fatty acids are called omega-3 and omega-6. These two fatty acids are used by the cells to help protect the cells when they are invaded by pathogens, for they start the chemical cascade to inflammation. When an invader such as a virus or bacteria goes beyond the digestive tract, the immune system reacts by sending three types of white blood cells, T-cells, B-cells, cytokines, and immunoglobins, antibodies, and complement proteins to attack and destroy. When the immune cells attack the antigens, a fight to the death occurs. This fight or war results in what medical researchers call "inflammation."

Inflammation protects the body from harmful results that antigens or pathogens can produce. The body uses inflammation to tell you that something is going wrong with your body. It tells you through three symptoms: swelling, redness, and pain. Inflammation can be a "good thing" or a "bad thing." The good is that it warns you of a problem or dysfunction within the body and that you need to quickly find a remedy or this dysfunction might get worse. It can also be a bad thing because inflammation might attack the body without any physiological reason. This type of inflammation is called "autoimmune disease." This means the body will attack itself for no apparent reason. And the pain can be excruciating. The disease of arthritis can be a perfect example of this type of inflammation.

The typical answer in our culture for inflammation is to combat inflammation with drug therapy. Unfortunately, some drugs have side effects that can cause other medical problems. For example, aspirin can significantly reduce pain by blocking or inhibiting prostaglandins from being released by the cell, which calls the immune system into action. This blocking or inhibiting action stops the pain. Stopping the pain makes everyone happy. However, taking too many aspirins can cause significant bleeding within the digestive system. Other drugs like ibuprofen, acetaminophen, Celebrex, and Singulair have also reported severe side effects.

The better answer to inflammation is to consume foods that don't contain arachidonic acid (AA). I feel the main culprit to inflammation is arachidonic acid. If we reduce AA production, we can stop the causes of inflammation.

Research has found that foods which are high in arachidonic acids are meats, dairy products, palm oil, store bought egg yolk—AA is especially high in farm-raised (not free range) animals. Farm-raised (not free range) animals such as fish, chicken, and beef are fed processed or genetically altered wheat, corn, and soy. Animals fed this way produce significantly higher amounts of AA within their bodies. When we consume these animals, we also consume a much greater amount of AA.

Let's examine salmon, which is one of the most nutritious foods that we can find. Analysis of farm-raised salmon (fed processed grain) revealed that 4 ounces of the fish contained 1325 milligrams of arachidonic acid. Analysis of wild salmon caught in oceans revealed 175 milligrams of arachidonic acid. The increase from farm-raised to wild was over 7:1. The increase from farm-raised chicken compared to free range was 4:1. The increase from farm-raised beef compared to grass fed beef was 2:1. The explanation for the lower increase in farmed raised beef was traced to the fact that farm-raised cattle were allowed to eat grass after their consumption of processed grain.

As you can see, we are harming our health by the way we are feeding our animals. I do want to point out that not all farm-raised animals are fed processed or genetically modified grain. Some are fed unprocessed grain and do not exhibit the above drastic results. You have to find out which way they are fed if you want to reduce arachidonic acid.

Comparison of Arachidonic Acid (AA) in Animal Protein

Farmed Conventional	AA	Natural—Free Range Feeding
Chicken	4 x as much as	Free Ranged Chicken
Fish	7 x as much as	Wild Fish
Beef	2 x as much as	Grass Fed Beef
Turkey	4 x as much as	Wild Turkey
Pork	5 x as much as	Wild Pork
Lamb	2 x as much as	Grass Fed Lamb

Couey's Six-Week Challenge

To help you overcome or reduce the pain associated with inflammation, I have devised a three-fold challenge for you to follow. Many of my clients have reported significant reduction in their pain.

1. *We must reduce the arachidonic acid in our bodies.* The following recommendations

must be strictly followed for six weeks if desired results are to be made.

a. No meat: This includes beef, chicken, turkey, pork, and lamb

b. No dairy: This includes milk, butter, cheese, and yogurt

c. No palm oil: Palm oil is high in foods that are crispy. Such as all types of chips and crackers.

d. No eggs

e. No farm-raised animals

2. The ratio of omega-6s to omega-3s should be 1:1 or no greater than 4:1.

Most Americans are eating fifty times more omega-6s than omega-3s. This means the omega-6s are breaking down into large amounts of arachidonic acid (see fig. 1.2). To counteract this, we must consume large amounts of foods that contain omega-3s. Foods that are high in omega-3s are raw nuts, flaxseed, and wild fish.

During Couey's Challenge you must consume *raw* nuts such as walnuts, almonds, cashews, pecans, and peanuts. Raw nuts are not roasted or salted. Sprinkle these raw nuts on salads and cereals. Snack on them between meals when necessary. Flaxseed and flaxseed oil are very high in omega-3's. Use flaxseed often in your diet.

Eating wild fish will help you consume omega-3s, which will help you balance the ratio to omega-6s. There are three types of fish that should be avoided. They are tilapia, grouper, and catfish. These fish are usually farmed or have very little omega-3s in them. Wild fish such as salmon, halibut, sardines, tuna, sea bass, orange roughy, mahi mahi, trout, and snapper contain large amounts of omega-3s. I recommend that you consume the above wild fish at least three to five times per week. Eating these fish baked or grilled would also help cut down on calories if you have a weight issue.

As you can see, the purpose of Couey's Challenge is to change the chemistry in the cell. We are trying to reduce arachidonic acid by cutting down on foods that contain omega-6s. Conversely, we are also trying to add omega-3s, which should help get the ratio from 50:1 to less than 4:1.

If we can change the abnormal chemistry in the cell to a more normal chemistry, then the cell will not send out messages for the immune system to attack it, thus preventing inflammation.

3. *Glycemic Index: The third challenge we face is to eat foods that are low on the glycemic index.* The glycemic index shows your glucose or sugar level. The glucose level is the most monitored physiological function in the human body. The reason for

this is because glucose is the brain's food. The human brain needs approximately 140 grams of glucose a day. It needs this glucose in a steady amount. If you consume too much glucose or too little glucose, then the brain reacts, causing what is known as "brain fog." You will have trouble remembering, have very little energy, and you will become sleepy and lethargic.

Most medical authorities recommend that the glucose level remains between 70 milligrams to 120 milligrams. If your glucose level exceeds 120 milligrams or drops below 70 milligrams, then the brain demands help from the pancreas to help balance the glucose between those parameters. The pancreas will release insulin if the glucose level goes too high. It does this to bring the glucose level back to within normal range. If the glucose level drops too low, then the pancreas will release glucagon which causes the glucose level to rise to normal levels.

If you eat foods that are high on the glycemic index, then the glucose level may rise very quickly to 200 milligrams or higher. This causes the pancreas to release large amounts of insulin, which can cause the glucose level to drop quickly to 50 milligrams or below. This condition is called hypoglycemia.

The symptoms of hypoglycemia:
- Brain fog
- Coma
- Death may occur
- Headaches
- Loss of consciousness
- Severe tiredness
- Shaking

It has been estimated that approximately 100 million Americans experience a mild to severe form of hypoglycemia.

Many medical authorities believe that some forms of hypoglycemia can be a predisposition to diabetes. Americans lead the world in the number of diabetics. We have 100 million with pre-diabetes. Diabetes can affect your heart, kidneys, and circulation to the legs and eyes. Diabetes is the leading cause of amputations and blindness in America. Many times adult-onset diabetes can be reversed or prevented by diet and exercise. Preventing this horrible disease should be a priority for every person in America.

Foods high on the glycemic index:

Let's get back to Couey's Challenge and the prevention of inflammation. When insulin level goes up quickly, it stimulates enzymes to produce more arachidonic acid and thus inflammation. We should eat foods that are low on the glycemic index, which will prevent high insulin release by the pancreas. Remember, eating foods high on the glycemic index will cause a quick rise in the glucose level and cause a high insulin response.

Foods high on the glycemic index include:

- Processed foods
- Foods containing white flour
- Foods containing white sugar or corn syrup
- Candy
- Baked desserts—pies, cakes, cookies, etc.
- White Rice
- Baked breads
- White potatoes

What should you eat?

After you have completed the six-week Couey Challenge, the following food plan should be a good guideline to follow the rest of your life. It will definitely keep your arachidonic acid at a normal level, which will protect you from run-away inflammation.

1. *Eat whole grains.*
   a. Whole grain bread—I recommend Ezekiel bread, if available. Otherwise, learn to mill your own wheat and make all your own bread products. Your health will increase rapidly. Watch out for the label "whole wheat bread," for it is processed. The producers just didn't bleach the endoderm white. Don't let the color of the bread fool you. The label must read "whole grain wheat bread." Put some almond or cashew butter on the bread. You can also use all-natural fruit jelly or jam, if you prefer.
   b. Whole grain cereals: Cheerios, Wheat Chex, and Bran Chex are a good example of a whole grain cereal. I recommend putting soymilk, rice milk, or almond milk on your cereal instead of pasteurized milk. Select various types of berries, such as blueberries, strawberries, raspberries, goji berries, or acai berries and sprinkle them liberally on your cereal.
   c. Whole grain oats—Put some raw nuts or fruit on your oatmeal. I recommend that you use stevia as a sweetener, for it is made from an herb.

    d.   Whole grain pasta—Use a vegetable- or fruit-based sauce. Don't forget to use grass-fed beef or free-range chicken for your meat sauce.

    e.   Brown rice—think of brown rice as a whole grain.

2.   *Eat legumes.*

Eat large amounts of beans and peas. Always try to eat them as fresh as possible. Frozen is alright, but watch out for legumes in cans. Sometimes the food producers add many preservatives.

3.   *Eat tubers.*

Tubers are foods that are grown under the ground.

    a.   Eat sweet potatoes or new red potatoes instead of white potatoes. These potatoes cause digestive enzymes to slowly break the carbohydrate into glucose, which causes a lower insulin response.

    b.   Other tubers, such as onions, carrots, garlic, turnips, beets, and radishes, are excellent sources of nutrition.

4.   *Eat any type of fruit.*

You should try to eat at least one source of fruit every day. If you are diabetic, then you may have to reduce or eliminate the following fruit because of their high glycemic effect: pineapple, watermelon, mangos, kiwi, and bananas.

5.   *Eat any type of vegetable.*

All varieties of vegetables are an excellent source of nutrition. I feel you should eat at least five servings a day with two vegetables being cruciferous. Eating these vegetables raw in a salad would also add enzymes to your nutrition.

6.   *Eat wild fish.*

Wild fish contains high sources of omega-3 fatty acids, which can help keep the production of arachidonic acid at a low level.

7.   *Eat grass fed beef.*

Grass fed beef has much lower levels of arachidonic acid in it, which helps control inflammation. Beef that is fed processed or genetically engineered corn, soy, and grain has a much higher arachidonic acid level, which promotes inflammation.

8.   *Eat free range chicken and turkey.*

Chickens and turkeys that are allowed to eat in natural outdoor settings have far less arachidonic acid present in them.

9.   *Eat dairy products in moderation.*

Americans are consuming too many dairy products that are pasteurized and homogenized or altered. We should consume raw milk products.

10. *Drink smoothies that are made from natural fruits and vegetables.*

You can make a delicious combination of fruits and vegetables with a blender.

Following the above recommendations will provide your cells with the necessary twenty-seven chemical elements in their proper amounts so that the cells can function at their highest performance. This means you can be protected against many types of inflammatory diseases or you can better fight the inflammation that you already have.

THYROID

The thyroid is a gland that follows instructions well. When told to do so, it will produce hormones. These hormones will complete many tasks, including providing the calories that are needed to sustain life while you are resting, controlling calcium in your blood, and controlling normal growth and development.

Factors that affect the thyroid and its ability to perform include:

- Allergies
- Chemical toxins
- Drug reactions
- Minerals
- Protein
- Radiation
- Stress
- Viruses

The thyroid controls how quickly the body burns calories and uses energy by secreting two main temperature-regulating hormones: triodothyronine (T3) and thyroxin (T4). The thyroid cells are the only ones capable of absorbing iodine. They combine iodine with the amino acid tyrosine to create the thyroid hormones.

An overproduction of the hormones is called "*hyper*thyroidism," resulting in an overactive metabolic state. Symptoms of hyperthyroidism include intolerance to heat, hair and weight loss, nervousness, less frequent menstruation, rapid heartbeat, and irritability.

"*Hypo*thyroidism" is an underproduction of the thyroid hormone and is more common. Symptoms of Hypothyroidism include:

- Chronic Fatigue
- Inability to tolerate cold/Low body temperature
- Painful or heavy premenstrual periods
- Hair loss
- Hoarseness
- Depression
- Dry and brittle nails

- Easy weight gain
- Elevated cholesterol
- Fertility problems
- Muscle weakness or cramps
- Recurring infections
- Constipation
- Goiter

The most effective way to determine how well your thyroid is functioning is to take the resting early morning under-arm temperature with a thermometer. Daily readings should maintain between 97.6 and 99.2° F. Since temperatures will vary with a women's cycle, it is best to do this for several weeks to see if fluctuations are due to menstruation and not the thyroid.

Recommendations:

- Follow God's plan for a healthy lifestyle: avoid processed food, drink enough distilled water, begin a moderate exercise program, and get plenty of rest.
- Reduce or eliminate alcohol, caffeine, and sugars.
- Avoid fluoride and chlorine (found in tap water and toothpaste), as these are chemically related to iodine, blocking the iodine receptors in the thyroid gland and leading to reduced hormone production.
- The conventional treatment for hypothyroidism is usually a prescription for a synthetic thyroid hormone.
- Applying a progesterone cream (available at health food stores) is often helpful to thyroid function.
- A kelp supplement may also be helpful, since it contains iodine.
- Do not self-diagnose or self-treat any issue. Please refer to a professional for testing and treatment.

OUR MENTAL HEALTH

And Jesus grew in wisdom…

Luke 2:52 NIV

Increasing our Mental Ability

DURING HIS LIFE, Jesus demonstrated scholarly growth and development many times. In Luke 2:47, Jesus, at age twelve, amazed even the scholarly priests with his knowledge of Old Testament Scripture. We should follow the example of Jesus. Know the scriptures. This is a result from spending considerable time in study and memorizing, which will in turn improve our mental capabilities to their fullest potential.

The prospective for our mental development is almost unlimited. For example, our brain contains approximately 30 billion cells, which are interconnected with each other. This means the possible interconnections are approximately 30 billion to the 30 billionth power. Scientists theorize that our brain could be stimulated properly to recall everything we have ever seen and heard from birth until the present. Yet everything we have experienced during our lifetime would comprise only about 10–15% of the brain's total potential.

Many people, including Christians, fail to cultivate their brain's mental promise. They have allowed their minds to become stagnant. They go to work, work at the same job every day, return home, and watch the same television programs. They get into the same everyday routine, and you know the result…they get bored. God has created in the brain tremendous capacity for mental development. It is up to you to develop this unlimited potential.

To learn effectively, a mental overload must be placed consistently on your mind. This overload should contribute positively, not negatively, to mental growth. Read educational books, watch television programs that increase knowledge, attend conferences to broaden your education; even taking up a new hobby can increase your brain's functioning power. Christian, avoid going stagnant. Do not be afraid or too lazy to learn about new areas of life. Develop the God-given potential by consistently overloading your mind with positive educational thoughts.

FOUR MAIN CAUSES FOR SLEEPING DISORDERS

The sleep of a working man is pleasant.

Ecclesiastes 5:12

1. *Hormonal Imbalance*

The following hormonal deficiencies are common causes of the inability to sleep:

- Deficiency of progesterone
- Estrogen dominance over progesterone
- Low levels of estrogen after menopause
- Low levels of melatonin. *Caution: DO NOT* use a melatonin supplement unless your blood levels indicate you are *low*. Using melatonin when it is not needed can cause autoimmune disorders.
- Low levels of DHEA. *Caution: DO NOT* use DHEA unless your blood levels indicate you are *low*.

2. *Mineral Imbalance*

Lack of sleep is often due to lack of calcium and magnesium and an electrolyte imbalance (often a low level of potassium). Root vegetables, bananas, celery, alfalfa, and a good natural endurance drink are good sources of potassium.

3. *Low Blood Sugar*

People who tend to be hypoglycemic can experience insomnia, or the inability to sleep through the night.

- Soy protein before bedtime is fabulous
- No simple carbohydrates at bedtime

4. *Stress*

Stress management is the key at every stage of life, but as we age the glands recover much more slowly from intense or chronic stress.

- Valerian is a muscle relaxant, and is very valuable to help reduce insomnia due to stress.
- Daily glandular nutrients are key; protein, B Complex, Vitamin C and Zinc

STRESS

He gives strength to the weary, and to him who lacks might He increases power. Though youths grow weary and tired and vigorous young men stumble badly, Yet those who wait for the Lord will gain new strength; They will mount up with wings like eagles, They will run and not get tired, They will walk and not become weary.

Isaiah 40:29–31

Stress is the gap between the demands placed upon us and the strength we have to meet those demands. In our country, we are not dying of infectious diseases anymore. We are dying of lifestyle diseases—degenerative diseases, such as heart disease, cancer, and diabetes. Stress can bring about any one of these three diseases, even though a person is eating the right foods, exercising, and supplementing correctly. Stress, along with un-forgiveness, can destroy your health and the health of your family.

Causes of Stress:
- *Environment (external)*—noise, heat and cold, toxins, travel, jobs, family
- *Diet*—malnutrition, illness, being overweight, drugs, processed foods, medicine
- *Exercise*—lack of exercise can cause small amounts of stress seem monumental.
- *Attitude*—anger, resentment, envy, guilt, revenge, tension, anxiety, unforgiveness, fear of change, rejection, job loss, finances, home life, depression, love, joy, unrealistic expectations, low self-esteem, self criticism, perfectionism, and worry all affect our stress levels.

We cannot control all stress, but we can control how we react to stress. All ages have stress, and they are going to find their strength is gone to handle difficult situations. We need to remember, it is not a sin to be stressed or weary. Even Jesus was weary; he was tired. Jesus set an example of spending time in prayer to his Father, and so must we spend time in prayer to God, our Father.

As you serve and follow through with the demands placed on you, you can become stressed. As mentioned above, the difference between the necessities laid upon you and the strength to meet those duties is what causes stress.

Stress Warning Signs and Symptoms

Cognitive Symptoms:

- Memory problems
- Indecisiveness
- Inability to concentrate
- Trouble thinking clearly
- Poor judgment
- Seeing only the negative
- Anxious or racing thoughts
- Constant worrying
- Loss of objectivity
- Fearful anticipation

Emotional Symptoms:

- Moodiness
- Agitation
- Restlessness
- Short temper
- Irritability, impatience
- Inability to relax
- Feeling tense and "on edge"
- Feeling overwhelmed
- Sense of loneliness and isolation
- Depression or general unhappiness

Physical Symptoms:

- Headaches or backaches
- Muscle tension and stiffness
- Diarrhea or constipation
- Nausea, dizziness
- Insomnia
- Chest pain, rapid heartbeat
- Weight gain or loss
- Skin breakouts (hives, eczema)
- Loss of sex drive
- Frequent colds

Behavioral Symptoms:

- Eating more or less
- Sleeping too much or too little
- Isolating yourself from others
- Procrastination, neglecting responsibilities
- Using alcohol, cigarettes, or drugs to relax
- Nervous habits (e.g. nail biting, pacing)
- Teeth grinding or jaw clenching
- Overdoing activities (e.g. exercising, shopping)
- Overreacting to unexpected problems
- Picking fights with others

Stress and Your Health

Many medical conditions are caused or exacerbated by stress, including:

- Asthma
- Autoimmune diseases
- Chronic pain
- Diabetes
- Heart disease
- Heartburn
- High blood pressure
- Infertility
- Irritable bowel syndrome
- Migraines
- Obesity
- PMS
- Skin problem
- Ulcers

Chemical Changes in the Body from Stress:

- Fight or flight—stress causes an increase in production of adrenaline and stress hormones, which causes a depletion of Vitamins B and C.
- Blood sugar rises—With Vitamin B depleted, the body is unable to convert sugar to energy; the pancreas becomes overworked to produce insulin to control the sugar. The pancreas collapses, which leads to hypoglycemia and diabetes.

- Heart begins pounding and lungs breathe faster—vitamin E is depleted to bring more oxygen to the cells.
- Muscles Tense—not enough calcium/magnesium to handle stress.
- Digestive and reproductive system shuts down—Food only partially digested, enzymes slow down, and food putrefies, colon sluggish, ulcers result. Prostate problems, impotency, PMS, endometriosis, fibroid tumors, menstrual problems, etc.

Stress Management:

Stress management is the key at every stage of life, but as we age, the glands recover much more slowly from intense or chronic stress.

- Valerian is a muscle relaxant and is very valuable in helping to reduce insomnia due to stress.
- Daily glandular nutrients are key—protein, B-complex, vitamin C, and zinc.

Diet Necessary to Prepare for or Prevent Stress:

The diet for stress is no different than the diet we are studying throughout this entire manual and the Bible study. When we give our bodies a smorgasbord of high-quality protein, whole grains, and raw fruits and veggies, then our bodies will be better prepared to handle stress and recover quickly.

Supplements* Necessary to Allow Your Body to be Prepared and Recover Quickly from Stress:

- B-Complex
- Calcium/magnesium
- Herbs; ashwaganda, beta- sitosterol
- Multi-Vitamin
- Protein—high-quality soy protein
- Vitamin C
- Vitamin E
- Zinc—for skin problems

* Beware of products containing KAVA; this is associated with severe liver damage.

Childhood Stress Symptoms:

Everyone experiences stress, only some people are able to handle it better than others. Even children experience stress. Here are some signs of stress in children:

- Acting Out
- Bedwetting
- Changes in sleep patterns
- Difficulty learning and difficulty leaving you
- Drastic changes in school work
- Headaches
- Mood swings
- Stomach aches
- Symptoms in older children: lying, bullying, defying authority
- Symptoms young children : nightmares and hair twirling

Solutions for Stress in Children:

- Pray daily for your children. If you feel uncertain of how to do this, then understand that God just wants to know your heart, and the only words necessary are to tell him your need for his help in raising your kids. If you feel you want to understand this better, *The Power of a Praying Parent"* by Stormie Omartian and *Praying for Your Child* by Dr. Dobson are excellent resources to use.
- Proper Rest—a minimum of 8 hours sleep
- Nutrition—the guidelines in this manual will give everyone a body to cope better with and recover faster from stress.
- Good parenting—Make sure you spend time in the same room as your children. Give them time to talk to you without any pressure. Get on the floor and play with them. Be interested in them and their interests.
- Let them play creatively.
- Cut back on after school activities.
- Keep a journal of their behavior.
- Spend more time talking.
- Help them prepare for situations that may cause stress ahead of time. For example, talk about the doctor visit before you go.
- Some stress is normal. Let the child know it is OK to feel angry, scared, lonely, and anxious.

Do not fear, for I am with you; Do not anxiously look about you, for I am your God. I will strengthen you, surely I will help you, and surely I will uphold you with My righteous right hand. I am the Lord your God, who upholds your right hand, Who says to you, Do not fear, I will help you.

(Isaiah 41:10, 13)

Stretching Exercises to Reduce Muscle Tension

When we sit at a desk all day doing paper work or computer work, muscles contract for long periods of time, and we need to periodically stop and stretch those muscles to prevent tension.

1. *Neck Stretch*

Many of us hold a lot of tension in our neck muscles. Sit up in your chair. Put your right hand on top of your head and gently pull your head down toward your right shoulder. Put your left hand down at your side and lift your left hand so it is like a table and the fingers are pointing straight out from your left side. Feel the stretch along the side of your neck.

Now repeat on the other side. Put your left hand on top of your head and gently pull your head down toward your left shoulder. Put your right hand down at your side and lift your right hand so it is like a table and the fingers are pointing straight out from your right side. Feel the stretch along the side of your neck.

2. *Chest Stretch*

Most of us sit hunched over all day with our chest muscles contracted and our upper back stretched. We want to stretch those chest muscles and contract the back.

Stretch your arms in front of you with your thumbs touching side by side. Now, open your arms out to the side and as far back as you can go. Bring your shoulders down and back. This is stretching the deltoids and chest.

3. *Lower Back Stretch*

Sitting in your chair, cross your right leg over your left leg. Put your left hand on your right leg and grab the back of your chair with your right hand. Pull gently and square your shoulders against the chair. This is going to give you a nice stretch to the lower back. Repeat on the other side.

4. *7–1 Stretch*

Sitting in your chair, extend your right leg out in front of you. Reach with the left arm for the ball of your foot and pull. Bend your leg if you need to. This stretches the deltoid muscles in your shoulders, the neck, lower back, hamstring, and calf and heel chord.

Now repeat with the left leg out in front of you. Reach with the right arm for the ball of your foot and pull.

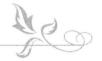

OUR SPIRITUAL HEALTH

And Jesus grew in…favor with God.

Luke 2:52

JESUS LEARNED EARLY in life about the tremendous potential given to him for developing a close relationship. His close relationship with God is one we should try to duplicate.

Many Christians are unaware of the resources that God has provided for leading a rich and exciting life. The untapped potential lies within our grasp, yet we lead a mediocre, rollercoaster existence of occasional mountaintop experiences followed by slides back into the same rut. A few, having never experienced anything else, conclude this must be the normal Christian life. But Jesus came so that believers might have the "abundant" life (John 10:10). Abundant living is not all "peaches-and-cream" experiences. But if we are willing to make the investment, God will lead us into fulfillment and adventure with himself.

Guidelines for spiritual growth:

Rely on God's Resources and Personal Effort. The purpose of growing in Christ is to reflect his character to others and to minister to them that they may come to know him. According to the Bible, Christians do not grow just by their own strength but by the actions of God's Spirit within them. It is the believer's responsibility to spend time and energy fulfilling God's requirements for growth (Eph. 4–6). Frantic efforts to develop spiritual wholeness or a lackadaisical "leave all the rest to God" attitude do not produce growth. We as Christians are called both to rely on God's resources and to respond in obedience to him.

Live in the Fullness of the Holy Spirit. All who commit their lives to Christ receive the Holy Spirit. However, many Christians still do not yield to him or rely on the resources he brings into their lives. Through ignorance or rebellion, they miss the abundant life Christ promised and enter a cycle of frustration and depression.

If we are to live in the fullness of the Holy Spirit, we must confess all known sin and accept God's cleansing by faith. Confession of all known, unremembered, or unknown sin brings cleansing from all unrighteousness (John 1:9). This will bring a feeling of peace and freedom to your life.

Another way to live in the fullness of the Holy Spirit is to turn over all areas of our lives to Jesus (Rom. 12:1–2). Many Christians are afraid to totally yield their lives to Christ. They have pet sins they desire to retain. Or, they fear God will cheat them out of a really full life if they submit to him. We must realize that God intends what is best for us (Jer. 29:11). God desires we spend our lives on things of everlasting value, not on impressive and attractive things the world offers us. If you want to really live life, then yield your life in its entirety to his control, asking him to fill you and take charge. With the help of His power, commit yourself to break with those things displeasing to Him and to develop in your life those patterns honoring Him.

Grow in Personal Knowledge of God. In order to get to know God, you must spend time with him and learn more about him. Develop a daily time with God. Personal relationships demand personal time together. Even Jesus found it necessary to set aside a special time for communication with the Father (Mark 1:35). Our time with God before the day starts will set the tone for the entire day. Yield to God in prayer for control and filling of your life. Express thanks and praise to him. Pray over matters affecting you daily.

Gain a practical grasp of God's Word. An understanding of the Bible will help you develop a closer relationship with God. One of the major reasons many Christians do not live a fuller life is their ignorance of biblical teachings. Unawareness of its guidelines on right and wrong causes you to fall into sin and waste. Listening, reading, studying, and meditating are excellent methods to achieve knowledge of God and obedience of his way.

Use Opportunities to Minister to Others. A key part of God's plan for our growth is service. What we receive from him, he desires we minister to others. We can minister to others about God's grace by becoming a part of a fellowship of Christians. When you join a local church you will have the opportunity to help others and be helped by them as they teach and encourage you. Learn to share Christ with others around you. If you ask him to, and yield to him, God will use you to share the good news about Christ.

Utilize God's resources (his promises, his Spirit, his Word, and his church) for spiritual growth. Proper use of these resources will help you to develop into the total person.

You may benefit from the *Treasures of Healthy Living Bible Study*. The spiritual part of the equation for our total health represents a small part of this book, but the *Treasures of Healthy Living Bible Study* takes the reader through twelve weeks of in-depth study into the Old and New Testament. The reader will discover many treasures found in God's Word to unlock the full potential of health. The practical weekly applications give assistance to understand and implement changes in a fun way. The treasure hunt includes topics such as fasting, stress, unforgiveness, Scripture memory, joy, laughter, and relationships. All these coupled with the learning about foods makes this study a long-treasured delight.

PRAYER AND FASTING

There are no concrete commandments concerning fasting in the Bible. There is not much explanation for the purpose of fasting either. Most of what we learn is by precedent and gleaning from the context of the various texts that mention fasting.

The most powerful word from God we have concerning fasting is in Mark 9:14– 29. Jesus refers to a particular demonic stronghold that could be mastered only through "prayer and fasting." This gives us our basis for belief of fasting. When done for the right reasons, it can aid our prayer time as we focus on a particularly difficult situation.

Because God's Word leaves us a good bit of leeway when it comes to fasting, here are a few thoughts on the subject that are gleaned from Scripture and fasting experiences. Let me challenge you to delve into the full study of fasting in the *Treasures of Healthy Living Bible Study*.

Purpose:

One benefit fasting brings to our prayer time is the constant reminder from our bodies to stay in an attitude of special prayer. Every time our bodies remind us that we haven't eaten, we are reminded of our prayer need.

Another aspect of fasting with prayer is that the very act of fasting puts our prayers above even the natural need to eat.

Duration:

Traditionally fasts go from evening to evening. Length can certainly be adjusted, but should be determined before the fast actually begins. If fast is done in conjunction with others, a "length of fast" can be set by the group.

What Constitutes a "Fast"?

Some go without food or water. I think this is a bit extreme. "Water only" is a reasonable choice. (This should not preclude a breath mint for the sake of others!) Another reasonable choice is liquids only. This is especially good for those taking medicine and people who must put in a full work day. This could include milk, broth, and juice, but I would leave off the "milkshake."

Some eat only fruit and vegetables. This may negate many of the benefits of fasting, but could be of some use.

Activity While Fasting

It would be great to be free from all others activities so the time could be devoted exclusively to prayer. Usually though, most normal activities are continued with the exception of activities that would be strictly for pleasure.

Prayers are voiced and/or offered silently throughout the day as circumstances permit. Special segments of time should be allotted for nothing but prayer.

Who should know?

Let as few people as possible know besides the participants. Family, close friends and people you normally eat with may need to be told. (See Matthew 6:16–18.)

Keep in mind!

This is not a weight-loss effort. Do not weigh yourself before starting or after finishing.

Once you commit to the fast (in your own heart), do not break it. Fasting should be done only by those who are spiritually mature enough to have rule over their desires.

This is not a secret weapon to be drawn on any situation we don't like. God retains His sovereignty and can still answer "yes, no, or wait." What we can know, assuming we are living in the center of His will, is if we don't receive, it won't be because we didn't ask!

Spiritual Benefits of Fasting

1. To receive divine guidance, revelation, or an answer to a specific problem
2. To hear God better and to understand more fully His will for your life
3. To weaken the power of the adversary (some refer to fasting as getting a "holy oiling" and because of it, the world, the flesh, and the devil can't hold on to you. You slip right through their clutches into freedom, but there is no Scriptural reference for this view point. ☺)
4. To cope with present monumental difficulties
5. To have freedom from bondage
6. To establish a position of spiritual strength and dominion
7. To be released from heavy burdens (your or others')
8. To break through a depression

9. To invite the Lord to create in you a clean heart and renew a right spirit

10. To seek God's face and have a closer walk with Him

11. To seek the Lord when He is directing you to do something that you don't think you have the ability to do

12. To be free of evil or debilitating thoughts

13. To resist temptation

14. To be set free from everyday sins—pride, jealousy, resentment, gluttony, gossiping, etc.

15. To help you when you are feeling confused

16. To help you when life seems out of control

17. To humble yourself

18. To break the lusting of the flesh after anything

19. To gain strength

20. To invite God's power to flow through you more mightily

Physical Benefits of Fasting

1. Cleansing process, detoxification

2. Rest for all of our bodies' systems and a time of new cell growth

3. Reverses or slows aging process

4. Clearer thinking, emotional stability

5. Improved overall appearance

6. Added strength

7. Contributes toward weight loss

8. Eliminates cravings

9. Improves immune system

10. Improves digestion

Biblical References for Fasting

2 Samuel 3:35–36   2 Samuel 12:1–23

Matthew 6:16   1 Samuel 7:6

Matthew 4:23; 6:16–18   Exodus 34:28

Joel 1:14; 2:12–14

Isaiah 58:1–7

Act 10:1–36; 13:3; 14:21–23

Matthew 17:21

Jeremiah 14:10–12

Ezra 8:21–23

Nehemiah 9:1–3

Esther 4; 9:31

Luke 18:12

Psalm 109:24

Daniel 1:12–16

2 Chronicles 20:14

1 Corinthians 7:3–5

Jonah 3:5–8

FASTING TRACK SHEET AND PRAYER JOURNAL

Return to Me with all your heart and with fasting, weeping and mourning; and rend your heart and not your garments. Now return to the Lord your God for He is gracious and compassionate, slow to anger, abounding in loving kindness.

(Joel 2:12–13)

Date for fast to begin _____ Length of fast _____

3 days prior: Eat only foods God created in their purest, most natural form possible. This would mean avoiding processed food as much as possible.

Day _____ Type of fast for this day _____

Keep a log of how you are feeling, what you are consuming (food, liquid), and what Bible verses you spent time meditating on.

_____

_____

_____

_____

_____

_____

_____

_____

_____

_____

_____

_____

_____

_____

_____

Commit your works to the Lord, and your plans will be established.

~Proverbs 16:3

HEALTHY FAMILY

FAMILY CAN BE the most treasured keepsake. Keeping them healthy should be our utmost priority. This information will be a guide toward better choices in regards to each family member. Keep in mind what you have already learned in "Nuts about Nutrition," combine that with tasty recipes from the *Healthy Treasures Cookbook*, and you have a winning combination for years of great health and wonderful experiences for your family.

CHILDREN'S HEALTH

Hold on to instruction, do not let it go: guard it well…listen closely to my words…for they are life to those who find them and health to a man's whole body.

Proverbs 4:13, 20, 22

Allergies, Asthma, Digestive Disturbances—reflux, diarrhea, constipation, Irritable bowel syndrome—Crohn's disease, ADD, ADHD, Obesity, Depression, Emotional Disorders, Behavioral Disturbances, and Cardiovascular Disease are *all increasing at alarming rates in our children*!

Nutrient Deficiencies in Children

Deficient Nutrient	*Symptoms from Deficiency*	
1. Iron	Fatigue	Weakness
	Headaches	Pallor
	Listlessness	Irritable
	Learning disabilities	Anorexia

2. Vitamin C

Aversion to work   Hysteria
Depression   Listlessness
Weakness   Hypoglycemia
Social introversion   Fatigue

3. Magnesium

Apathy   Hyperirritability
Personality changes   Crave chocolate and sweets

4. Zinc

Poor appetite   Irritability
Failure to grow   Mental lethargy
Emotional disorders

5. B-Complex

Confusion   Poor coordination
Depressed appetite   Irritable
Sleep disorders   Fatigue
Generally miserable (whiner)
Depression   Agitation
Memory loss   Headaches
Emotional instability   Sleeplessness

6. Calcium/Magnesium

Abdominal pain   Muscle spasms
Bed-wetting   Fatigue
Headaches   Restlessness
Hyperactivity   Twitches
Irritability   Teeth-grinding/night
Poor sleeping habits
Pins and needles sensation on skin

7. Food Allergies

Abdominal pain   Excessive fatigue
Aggression   Glazed look
Bags/wrinkles under eyes   Hives
Bloating   Hyperactivity
Leg aches   Red earlobes
Dark eye circles   Red cheeks
Depression   Dry skin
Eczema   Wiggly/restless legs
Chronic ear, chest, sinus infections
Temper tantrums, whining, screaming

What is Lacking in Your Child's Diet?

As you can see from the list of deficiencies, we have a problem on our hands, but where did the problem originate? There are three primary reasons: the first is our food, the second is our lifestyle and the third is our responsibility as parents.

Our Food

Do you have a picky eater? For many parents this is their main problem but there are more factors contributing to the diet our children consume. Our food today is not what it used to be. Most of what we eat today is processed, sugar-laden, nutrient-deficient, chemical-loaded, and damaging to our bodies.

- National dietary surveys showed our children's diets fell short in the intake of many critical nutrients (as listed above).
- The New York Schoolchildren Survey reports 25% of the children surveyed had not eaten any fruits or vegetables in the past 24 hours.
- There is a calcium crisis in this country that has been exacerbated by the increased consumption of carbonated beverages, which interferes with calcium absorption.
- Studies show that 1 in every 13 children have asthma.
- Our meats are injected with antibiotics and hormones, while our fruits and vegetables are loaded and grown with pesticides and herbicides.
- Over 60,000 additives (artificial colors, artificial flavors, preservatives, sweeteners, etc.) are processed into the food, mostly for cosmetic reasons and preservation, not for nutrition.

Our Lifestyle

Our lifestyles make it difficult to eat well. We eat on the run. We need to take time to rest, relax, and plan healthy meals. We let TV influence our food choices along with the school lunch menus. As parents, we are responsible for the food our children eat, whether it is in our homes, while we are out, or while they are at school. This is an area of their lives we need to make a priority with healthy choices. The list of children's deficiencies could be partially and sometimes totally eliminated if the environment, food, and lifestyle were improved.

Dinner time is designed to be a time of sharing, fellowship, enjoying each other, and getting to know the family. This is a time to develop good eating habits for future optimal health. Many degenerative diseases children are now having at a young age are shown to decrease with improved changes in thinking, eating, and living habits.

Take time to fly a kite with your children; enjoy their lives, and let them enjoy yours.

Our Responsibility

There is a popularly quoted book written by a politician who says "It takes a village to raise a child". I totally disagree with this statement. The reason our children are having so many problems is that we have given our responsibility over to so many other people and organizations that we are not the ones raising our children anymore. The bottom line is that as parents we know foremost what is best for our kids and as Christian parents we have an excellent guide book to give us the answers we need. Meeting our kids' health needs is going to begin in the home with healthy meals, healthy relationships and spiritual leadership. This is our responsibility and we need to hold on to that with a grip like a one year old learning to walk. The best part of this responsibility is that we get to rejoice in the results of our time spent on this investment into our kids' lives.

Food Guide Pyramid Recommendations for Children

Recommended Number of Daily Servings by Age Group

FOOD GROUP	TODDLERS	CHILDREN	TEENS
Grains	6	9	11
Fruits	2	3	4
Vegetables	3	4	5
Protein	2	2	2–3
Dairy	2	2	2–3

Toxins in Our Environment[55]

Our children are being exposed to excessive amounts of toxins in the food they eat, the water they drink, the air they breathe, and in the environment in which they live. As parents, we need to become proactive and lobby against the use of dangerous pesticides and chemicals in this country. At the same time, we need to do everything we can to eliminate toxins in our homes and in the schools our children attend.

- According to the Children's Cancer Group Epidemiology Program, children are 5–6 times more likely to develop leukemia and brain cancer if their families use pesticides at home.
- Most of the increase in leukemia rates in the past 20 years has been in a kind of cancer called acute lymphoblastic leukemia (ALL). A recent study in the American Journal of Public Health reported an association between household chemicals and ALL.

- Cancer is the leading cause of disease-related deaths in children under the age of 20 (from the Centers for Disease Control and Prevention). Every year, about 12,400 children and teens under the age of 20 are diagnosed with cancer.
- The EPA states: "There are thousands of toxic chemical compounds in use today. New chemicals are developed each year and many of these can enter and contaminate both surface and underground water. In large amounts some of these chemicals found in drinking water could cause cancer, mutations, and birth defects."

Our Children's Immune Systems

One of our most important jobs as parents is to help our children develop healthy immune systems. The key to remember is that nutrition gained in childhood is a gift that lasts a lifetime. Children have a remarkable ability to heal themselves, especially if their immune systems are strong and healthy.

How the Immune System Works:

The immune system is made up of an army of special white blood cells, T-cells and B-cells, which are ready to go to war at a moment's notice. These special cells attack and destroy anything that invades the body or threatens it from without or within, including bacteria, viruses, and cancer.

If your immune system is working perfectly, then it should not attack anything considered healthy to your body, including "you." However, sometimes a person's immune system responds to harmless or useful substances as if they were the enemy. This is what happens in the case of allergies. To understand this better, read the information on "Leaky Gut" in this manual.

The immune system can be challenged by sugar, Candida, and antibiotics. To know if your child suffers from a Candida problem, there are three resources: "Candida" (in this manual), Candida Questionnaire (Designed Healthy Living Web site), and Nutritional Deficiency (Designed Healthy Living Web site). All of these tools can assist you in knowing if your child is dealing with a Candida issue.

Note that sugar in the diet can cause a deficiency in important vitamins and minerals. Sugar can also cause a rise in blood sugar and lead to diabetes.

Vicious Cycle of Antibiotics and Candid

Steps for Improving Your Child's Health

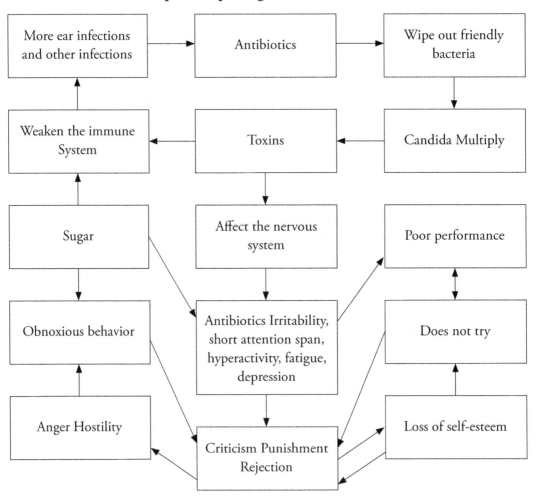

This vicious cycle can be unending if the same inputs are not removed. As you can see, getting rid of sugar in the diet is a positive step each parent can take. Getting rid of toxins and controlling the Candida is another step. Parents can take active roles in helping their children. The good news is this cycle can end if you seriously want change.

1. Create a loving and healthy home.

    *   Model the behavior you desire your children to have. You as the parent are the most influential person in your child's life.
    *   Involve the children in your choices of food, and discuss why you choose that for them. Make it a game to try new fruits and veggies.
    *   Try to create dips for your children to use with their new veggies.
    *   Encourage them to try new foods, but do this with love and gentleness. If you let them know and understand that you want to make everyone, including yourself, happier by being healthier, then they may join in with you on these new changes.
    *   Pray for your children. It is God's desire that your family is healthy, happy, and serving Him. Your prayers will bring about a change in your children that nagging will never accomplish. Also pray that your spouse will support you in this decision and will help with discipline when necessary.

Consider it all joy, my brethren, when you encounter various trials, knowing that the testing of your faith produces endurance. And let endurance have its perfect result, that you may be perfect and complete, lacking in nothing. But if any of you lacks wisdom, let him ask of God, who gives to all men generously and without reproach, and it will be given to him.

~James 1:2–5

2. *Follow a Healthy Food Plan.*

    *   Eat fresh, organic food whenever possible.
    *   Eat more veggies, raw or lightly cooked.
    *   Eat beans, lentils, seeds, nuts, and whole grains.
    *   Eat several servings of fresh fruit every day.
    *   Limit stimulants such as sugar, coffee, and tea.
    *   Avoid *all* artificial ingredients.
    *   Limit processed foods, including: refined bread, pasta, cakes, and cookies.
    *   Use meats and dairy products raised without antibiotics or hormones.
    *   Avoid "altered fats" found in margarine, heated oils, fast food, processed foods, and partially hydrogenated oils.
    *   Use organic butter and cold-pressed extra virgin olive oil.

3. *Remove all Toxins from the Home*

    *   Replace all toxic household cleaning and laundry products with safe, organic, and effective alternatives.

- Eliminate the toxins in your drinking water—lead, chlorine, gases, and chemicals—by using a high-quality water purifier or buying Reverse Osmosis purified water.
- Purify the air in your home and eliminate airborne contaminants such as mold, bacteria, viruses, and particulates with a high-quality air purifier.
- Prevent toxins from entering the skin by using safe, natural personal care products.

4. *Supplement by Age*

   Infants and Toddlers, 6 months to 2 years: Multi-Vitamin Infant powder and a probiotic as needed
   Ages 2–5: Chewable multivitamin, probiotic, chewable Vitamin C, Soy Protein
   Ages 5–18: Probiotic, Multi-Vitamin, Chewable calcium/magnesium, Vitamin C, Vitamin E, Protein

First Aid for Common Health Challenges

Cold or Flu:	Echinacea, Vita-C, Garlic, Alfalfa, and an immunity product
Nausea, Indigestion:	Ginger/Peppermint complex, Probiotic, Enzymes, Chewable calcium
Muscle Cramps:	Calcium/Magnesium, Extra magnesium, Valerian
Sleep Problems:	Valerian, Calcium/Magnesium
Constipation:	Make your own freshly milled bread, probiotics, fiber, or an herbal laxative

5. *Encourage Regular Exercise*

   - Spending twenty-five minutes outside every day is very important to the health of your child. It is surprising how they can even handle going out when it is freezing outside. Just bundle them up. The fresh air is worth it. It would be even better if you joined them outside.
   - Exercise will not only improve their physical health, but also it will improve their mental health.
   - Children should engage in vigorous, physical activity for at least thirty minutes each day to maintain cardiovascular fitness.
   - Plan family events to include hiking, bicycling, water activities, etc. Doing things as a family makes everyone have more fun. These events will create memories that will be long-treasured—much longer than sitting on the couch with a computer game in their hands and an IPOD in their ears!

MEN'S HEALTH

Liberty is to the collective body, what health is to every individual body. Without health no pleasure can be tasted by man; without liberty, no happiness can be enjoyed by society.

Thomas Jefferson

Liberty and health were joined together from the beginning of time in the Garden of Eden. When God set up plans for our well-being He had a purpose in mind to keep us healthy both spiritually and physically. This health was liberty to us. Today reaching this quality of health takes work and a mindset to 'make it happen'. As men, dads, and husbands you have the power in your leadership of the family to help bring this liberty to your family. To be the leader in eating healthy, exercising, and taking care of the body God has loaned you.

These next paragraphs are just a few highlighted topics to help you make better decisions and benefit from those decisions.

Creatine

Creatine works—it causes enlarged muscle mass! *But* the new muscle mass is weaker and tears and tires more easily. This puts you at risk of health problems:

1. How does this affect your heart muscle? Do you really want to create a larger heart that is weaker and tires more easily?

2. How does this affect your circulatory system? Do you really want to cause weakness in your veins, arteries, and capillaries to predispose yourself to a higher risk of aneurisms and strokes?

3. How does this affect your gastrointestinal system? Do you really want to cause weakness in your intestinal system, predisposing yourself to a higher risk of hernias?

4. How does this affect your prostate? Do you really want to cause it to enlarge and create urination problems?

Creatine use is a controversial issue. Many companies and Web sites state that it builds health, while others state the opposite. The truth is that creatine will require water from your bloodstream to build muscle mass. This means the individual requires more water during the use of this product and even more water while exercising. Many athletes have died from dehydration, and this can be prevented.

There are natural products available to build muscle in a healthy, balanced way. Search for companies that can prove their products are scientifically studied to build long-term health and not just short-term muscle. This is critical since we are planning on living for many years and not just past the next competition.

Remember, there are more muscles in your body than those in your legs and arms.

Prostate Health: What You Should Know

They say women live longer than men, and one reason might be women are more likely to go to the doctor when they have a problem. If that is true, and men do not want to go to the doctor for simple problems and instead wait till the problem is huge, then these pages on men's health will prove to be very beneficial. There are many self help plans listed to assist in preventing a diagnosis. However, these helps are *not* to replace appropriate medical screenings or exams. Read on, and learn how you can build and/or improve your health the natural way.

Prostate:

The prostate is the small gland, shaped like a donut, which surrounds the neck of the bladder and the urethra. Its major function is to contribute to seminal fluid. If it enlarges or swells, it can put pressure on the urethra, acting like a clamp. This condition is known as Benign Prostate Hyperplasia (BPH). Symptoms of early prostate cancer are similar to symptoms of BPH.

Problem:

The problem with the Prostate is certainly not new. It was affecting men in Egypt in the 15th century BC. According to Egyptian medical papyrus, they too suffered from enlarged prostate glands and sought relief by a variety of means.

In a young boy, the prostate is about the size of a marble. When the male hormones kick in, it grows to ping-pong ball size. Everything is fine until ages thirty to forty, when the prostate begins to grow again. This is normal and a nearly inescapable part of aging. The technical name for this growth is benign prostatic hyperplasia, or BPH. Nearly 60% of men by the age of forty-five have BPH. The problem is the prostate can grow too much, thereby pinching and narrowing the urethra, which causes a multitude of problems.

Three Main Problems:

1. *Prostate Cancer* is second only to lung cancer in men, and the rate is escalating. Men have the same risk of prostate cancer as women do for breast cancer. By age seventy-five, 50% of men develop prostate cancer. Symptoms are blood in the urine or reddish or pink urine, a burning sensation during urination, difficulty in starting urination, increasing frequency of arising at night to pass urine, and/or a high PSA blood test (PSA means Prostate Specific Antigen).

2. The PSA test is recommended every three years for men forty to sixty-five and annually for men over sixty-five. The results should be less than four.

3. *Prostatitis*: There are also two benign conditions affecting the prostate gland. One of them is prostatitis, an inflammation of the prostate that is usually caused by a fungal or bacterial infection. It can occur in men of any age, and generally responds to wise immune system treatment. Symptoms are pain between the scrotum and rectum, fever (infection often in the bladder), blood or pus in the urine, frequent urination accompanied by a burning sensation, and in advanced prostatitis, urination becomes more difficult.

4. *Benign Prostatic Hyperplasia* is the other non-malignant condition, which is the common prostatic problem and tends to impact men over the age of forty. Statistics show that it affects 60% of men from the age of forty to fifty-nine, and by age 80, 90% of men have problems. Symptoms are: having to strain to start urination, a weak urination stream, starting and stopping during urination, frequent urination night time urination, urgent signals, and dribbling after urination is complete.

How Do I Know if I Have These Problems?

There is a way to evaluate BPH symptoms in an organized way. Your doctor frequently uses a set of evaluation questions developed by the American Urological Association. Put a check in the box corresponding to the number of times you have the symptom described in the column. Then add up your total.

Symptoms over the past month:
0—Never
1—Less than 1 in 5 times
2—Less than half the time
3—About half the time
4—More than half the time
5—Almost always

	0	1	2	3	4	5

How often have you had a sensation of not emptying
your bladder completely after you finished urinating?

How often have you had to urinate again less than two
hours after you finished urinating?

How often have you found youstopped and started again
several times when you urinated?

How often have you found it difficult to postpone
urination?

How often have you had a weak urinary stream?

How often have you had to push or strain to begin
to urinate?

How many times did you typically get up to urinate
from the time you went to bed until the time you
woke up in the morning?

Your total: _____

Up to 7= Mild, 8–19= Moderate, 20–35= Severe

Why do you experience these problems?

Like any other gland, the prostate, in order to be healthy, needs to be nourished adequately, and zinc, B-complex, vitamin C, vitamin E with selenium, carotenoids, and soy protein are absolutely essential.

Dietary Recommendations:

Prostate cancer has been confirmed in the laboratory as being diet-related. Therefore, diet is important in the prevention and treatment of this disease.

- Maintain a whole food diet as much as possible.
- Drink half your body weight in ounces of water daily.
- Use cold-pressed oils, especially extra virgin olive oil, to obtain beneficial fatty acids.
- Consume more nuts, seeds, raw vegetables, fruits, fresh juices, dried beans, peas,

and brown rice. In particular, eat raw pumpkin seeds daily, as they are helpful in all prostate problems due to their high zinc content.

- Avoid refined carbohydrates, coffee, and strong tea, as these have been linked to prostate cancer.
- Cut way back on or eliminate alcoholic beverages, especially beer, which depletes the body's stores of zinc and vitamin B-6.
- Switch to organic sources of meat and dairy products to avoid excessive hormones that may have been fed to the animals. In general, limit your intake of meat and dairy.
- Avoid "trans-fatty acids" found in partially hydrogenated oils, margarine, processed food, and fast food, especially when oil is heated for long periods of time.

Lifestyle Recommendations:
- Exercise is really important. Walking is particularly beneficial, as it uses the muscles in the pelvic area, which helps improve circulation to all of the glands in that region of the body. Bicycle riding, however, is not recommended.
- Avoid exposure to very cold weather.
- Avoid Stress. Prostate cells are just as highly sensitive to emotional stress as the uterus, and it is very obvious the female hormonal cycle is greatly affected by stress.

Nutritional Supplements for Prostate Health[56]

Saw Palmetto is a unique herbal supplement that helps men maintain prostate health, proper urinary flow, and hormonal balance. Look for a supplement with a complex of nutrients: saw palmetto extract, pumpkin seed oil, beta-sitosterol, and soybeans, all of which have been found to have beneficial effects on the prostate.

- Many European studies have shown saw palmetto improves symptoms of benign prostate hyperplasia.
- Recently, the first randomized American clinical trial confirmed these results and showed this plant also reduced swelling in enlarged prostate tissue.
- In a study of 305 patients with mild to moderate symptoms of Benign Prostate Hyperplasia, supplementation with 160 milligrams of saw palmetto twice a day resulted in an 88% reduction of symptoms.
- An earlier, double-blind study found the following results after just one month of treatment: 47% decrease in nightly bathroom visits, 50% increase in urinary flow, and 42% reduction in residual urine.
- Saw palmetto works by inhibiting the enzyme, 5-alpha reductase, this converts

testosterone to its more active form, dihydrotestosterone (DHT), and it also blocks the binding of this hormone to receptor sites on the prostate.

- Saw Palmetto also increases the breakdown and excretion of DHT and helps stop the pain and inflammation associated with BPH.

Beta Sitosterol

- In a recent double-blind study of 100 men, those men taking 60 milligrams of beta sitosterol per day for six months had the following results: urinary flow increased 35% and residual urinary volume decreased by 54%.
- It has been hypothesized that beta sitosterol works by blocking hormone receptor sites on the prostate, thus preventing DHT from binding.

Pumpkin Seed Oil

- Complements and enhances the activity of saw palmetto
- Long history of use to prevent and treat prostate problems
- Active ingredients in pumpkin seed oil are fatty acids, one of which acts as a diuretic to help increase urinary flow.

Soybeans

- Genistein, an isoflavone in soy, has been found to halt the proliferation of prostate cancer cells and to prevent cancer growth in normal prostate cells.

Zinc

- Look for a tablet containing zinc gluconate.
- The prostate gland contains ten times more zinc than any other organ, and a lack of zinc has been shown to cause the prostate to enlarge.
- Researchers found the portion of the seminal fluid for which the prostate is responsible is high in zinc.
- In a study of men with BPH who were given zinc, blood levels of zinc did not increase but semen levels did increase with supplementation. When these men were given 150 milligrams of zinc in two months, 74% of them had a reduction in prostate size.
- Zinc works by inhibiting the production of the enzyme (5-alpha-reductase) that converts testosterone into its more active form, DHT.
- Normal amounts of zinc, up to 20 milligrams per day, have no effects on prostate enlargement, but medical experts agree that if you go over 80–100 milligrams per day, you are taking a risk with toxicity.

Vitamin E with Selenium

- Based on promising initial results, hospitals across the country have enrolled more than 32,000 healthy men in a study comparing the effects of vitamin E and the mineral selenium against sugar pills to determine if either or both can prevent prostate cancer.
- A major chemoprevention intervention trial in 1998 with 29,000 Finnish men found a 32% reduction in prostate cancer cases and a 41% decrease in cancer deaths with vitamin E supplementation.
- In a recent study, selenium supplementation (200mcg.day) was found to decrease the incidence of prostate cancer by more than 60%.
- In a large intervention trial for skin cancer, the surprise finding was that those people who took supplemental selenium had a 37% decrease in prostate, colorectal, and lung cancer, as well as a 50% reduction in cancer deaths.
- In a 1983 multi-institutional study, those patients treated with selenium had only about one-third as many prostate tumors as the patients receiving the placebo. In addition, there were not toxic effects of selenium supplementation.
- In a 1986 study, vitamin E was found to inhibit prostate cancer cell growth, and the inhibition was dose-dependent.
- In a Japanese study, low levels of vitamin E were associated with an increased risk of prostate cancer.

Essential Fatty Acid Supplements

- EPA, DHA, and GLA are critical intermediaries in the bio-chemical process whereby the essential fatty acids, linoleic acid, and linolenic acid are converted to GLA, DHA, and EPA, and then into prostaglandins—hormone-like substances that work to control and balance male hormones.
- In this country, this conversion process is often blocked by the presence of trans-fatty acids, found in margarine, fried and heated oil, fast food, and partially-hydrogenated oil—an ingredient in almost every processed food.
- Supplementation with GLA, EPA, and DHA helps restore this balance and has been found to result in a reduction of the symptoms associated with BPH and prostate cancer.

Self Help Programs
Men's Six Pack*

Bringing your health back to a normal energetic balance:

- Soy Protein
- Multi-Vitamin—including B- complex, vitamin C, and vitamin E

- Saw Palmetto
- Zinc
- Omega-3
- Probiotics

Prostatitis: Infection of the prostate

Traditional treatment involves antibiotics. These may successfully kill the infection, but weaken the immune system even more; so a man is far more prone to future infections. Herb and nutrient therapy is always a best choice to strengthen the body's own defense system.

- Echinacea compound
- Garlic
- Vitamin C 500 mg
- Pre and Pro biotic

Build the Immune System and nourish the Body:
- Soy Protein
- Daily vitamin/mineral
- Beta Carotene
- Natural Interferon

Prostate Cancer: is a malignancy where the cells multiply and spread. The four main causes of prostate cancer are:

1. Lack of Detoxification
2. Malnutrition (especially antioxidant vitamins)
3. Heated Oil consumption (trans-fatty acids)
4. Hormonal Imbalance

How Does a Cancer Develop?

A cancer cell develops when the chromosomes of a normal cell have been altered by "carcinogens." Lack of detoxification allows inappropriate substances to remain in the cellular tissue, and the cell stores more toxins than it can safely hold. This set up a vicious cycle:

- The accumulation of toxins reduces the cell's ability to detoxify, causing "intoxification."
- Intoxification causes irritation, interference with cellular function, and premature degeneration of the cellular tissue.

- This leads to damaged cellular DNA, which results in the abnormal growth and multiplication of the cell, what we know as "cancer."

Other causes of cancer are:

- Weak immune system
- Allergies
- Environmental toxins
- Stress
- Faulty digestive system
- Hormonal imbalance
- Trans-fatty acid consumption
- Parasites
- Genetics—but genetics do not have to express themselves unless the cellular environment becomes weakened.

Cancer is a major "Red Flag":

Cancer will occur in the weakest area of the body. It tells you your own immune system could not do its job. Traditional medical treatment involves surgery, chemo, or radiation. However, this *does not* address the root cause:

1. What caused the cancer to develop in the first place?
2. Why was your own immune system *too weak* to defend itself?

If you choose to do one of the recommended traditional treatments, *do not* presume that the cancer is gone and you can just move ahead in life. You have not addressed root causes. Where do you want the "Red Flag" to show up next? Take this wake-up call seriously, and implement the suggestions in this manual.

WOMEN'S HEALTH

Women's health is definitely misunderstood. Although many women feel like "roaring," as it says in Helen Reddy's song "I am Woman," others long to be the Proverbs 31 wife—"An excellent wife, who can find? For her worth is far above rubies." And in Proverbs 18:22 it says, "He who finds a wife finds a good thing, and obtains favor from the Lord." These verses typically sum up the person and wife we want to be today or in the future when we marry. The cycles of life and hormonal issues can be distracting and turn us into the monster that comes out of a cave at certain times of the month or certain years in our lives.

The information on this topic will assist you through these times in your life and restore a feeling of self-worth and happiness.

Introduction: Understanding Hormones

When a baby girl is born, she has all of the eggs she will ever have, between 350,000 and one million. During the fertile portion of her life she will begin to ripen approximately 1,000+ eggs each month at the beginning of each menstrual cycle. This happens as a response to the follicle stimulating hormone in the pituitary gland. There is a contest to see which one will be the egg of the month; usually only one wins, and the rest simply atrophy. When the follicles from the ovaries, which were stimulated by the pituitary gland, grow, they produce estrogen. Estrogen begins to thicken the lining of the uterus to receive the egg. The level of estrogen is at its highest on days 13–15 of your cycle. This high level of estrogen signals the pituitary gland to secrete LH hormone, which causes the follicle to rapidly mature and burst, releasing the egg. This is usually a day of discharge (milky mucous). The fallopian tube grasps the egg and begins to carry it to the uterus for possible fertilization.

Meanwhile, back at the ovary, the remainder of the ripened follicles transform into yet another gland—corpus luteum. This produces some estrogen and a lot of progesterone, which is the dominate hormone in the second half of the cycle. Progesterone prepares the womb for pregnancy by thickening the endometrium to a plush nursery for the fertilized egg. If the progesterone level is too low, a miscarriage can occur.

If no egg is present, the corpus luteum will disintegrate and shrink. This will cause the estrogen and progesterone to decline. When this happens, it causes the uterus to go into a spasm and contract to expel the lining. This is known as your period.

Endocrine System:

It requires a perfect balance of hormones to make everything happen properly. This means you must have healthy glands in the entire endocrine system.

The endocrine system is made of the pineal gland, pituitary gland, thyroid gland, parathyroid gland, thymus gland, adrenal gland, pancreas, and ovaries. There are over 100 hormones produced, including: testosterone, progesterone, estrogen (estrone, estroil, and estradiol), thyroxine, cortisone, and melatonin.

Recipe for the manufacturing of hormones:

- 22 amino acids
- Essential Fatty Acids
- Vitamins

- Minerals
- Probiotic

These hormones are released in the blood stream and bind to receptor sites on the cells like a lock and key. There are receptor sites in the cells of the vagina, bladder, breasts, skin, bones, arteries, heart, liver, and brain.

Cycles of Life

Puberty: begins at approximately age twelve. This is when follicles in the ovaries start to ripen. This will increase hormonal levels and lead to female body shape changes.

PMS: ages twelve to fifty, this pre-menstrual syndrome should not happen in a healthy woman. The common complaints are cramps, moodiness, pelvic pain, breast tenderness, nervous tension, fluid retention, bloating, and insomnia. One of the main reasons for PMS may be hormonal imbalance—excessive levels of estrogen and inadequate levels of progesterone—as well as sensitivity to fluctuating hormones. A vitamin/mineral deficiency and diet are main contributors to PMS, along with the body's inability to metabolize fatty acids.

Perimenopause: ages thirty-five to forty-nine, this is the beginning of a gradual reduction in reproductive hormones. This cycle may occur over several years. The storage of eggs is being depleted, and remaining eggs do not respond well to the command to be released. Some months you may release an egg and experience a heavy period, and the next month you may have no ovulation with little to nothing of a period. Perimenopause can last four months to five years, with many of the symptoms accompanying actual menopause. Even though a women's estrogen level may be dropping during this time, many women experience estrogen dominance because their progesterone is too low.

Menopause: it most commonly occurs between the ages of fifty and fifty-two; menopause is not an event, it is a process that takes place over a period of time as a woman "adjusts" to lower levels of estrogen. During this time, a women stops ovulating and her ovaries *decrease* the amount of hormones they produce. The average age for menopause is about fifty. This process is similar to puberty, in reverse.

Post menopause: A period of time ranging from three months to five years after the ability to bear children has ceased. Usually a lack of estrogen and possibility progesterone.

Nutritional Guidelines for PMS:

- Calcium/ Magnesium: Needed for insomnia, nervousness, muscle cramps, abdominal cramps, and pelvic pain. Research indicates women who have PMS may have lower levels of magnesium than women who do not have PMS. A deficiency in magnesium could account for several of the most common symptoms listed above. Many women who crave chocolate before their periods in fact may be craving magnesium. (Author's note—doesn't it sound better to crave chocolate than magnesium? Are you going to go make some magnesium brownies?)

- Dietary sources of magnesium are green leafy vegetables, whole grains, legumes, cereals, nuts, and seeds. Calcium and Magnesium work together. They should be taken together and in proper balance.
- B-Complex: Needed for the effective regulation of estrogen levels. When vitamin B supplies are insufficient, estrogen levels rise and PMS symptoms worsen. Increase in estrogen contributes to a further decrease in the B vitamins. They are useful in easing depression, headaches, dizziness, fatigue, irritability, mood swings, food cravings, and fluid retention. Dietary sources are eggs, whole grains, salmon, and brewer's yeast. Cooking, canning, processing, exposure to light and lengthy storage time may contribute to the destruction of the B-complex.
- Alfalfa: is a natural diuretic—it reduces fluid retention. It is also great with allergies, which can be bothersome for a PMS sufferer.
- Iron: If you tend to be low in iron, this is a good time to take extra. Not ferrous sulfate, this is the least absorbable. Ferrous fumarate is a good source.
- EPA: Take an Essential Fatty Acid from cold water fish. This is great for any inflammation.
- GLA: is great for many symptoms of PMS—moodiness, cramping, breast tenderness, poor libido, etc. Read about GLA in this manual.
- Vitamin E: helps balance hormonal irregularities. It is great for cystic conditions and tumors and improves circulation. Dietary sources include: cold pressed vegetable oils, all whole raw seeds, nuts, soybeans, and wheat germ oil.
- Vitamin C and Beta Carotene: for new tissue formation and antioxidant.
- Natural Interferon: new studies have proven natural interferon helps with PMS symptoms.
- Diet: follow the diet under the "Menopause" section.

Symptoms of Hormonal Imbalance

Estrogen Dominance: During childbearing years, women may experience hormonal imbalance symptoms, especially after ovulation and often caused by too much estrogen and not enough progesterone. The main reasons are:

a. inadequate nutrients to manufacture hormones (see recipe on previous page).
b. inadequate progesterone production due to stress, lack of rest, and interference from accumulated toxins in cellular tissue.

c. elevated estrogen caused by: xenoestrogens or xenobiotics (chemical from the environment that mimic estrogen in the body), usually 1,000 times the strength of human estrogen. (Read about this in detail under "Xenobiotics" in this manual).

- estrogen in food supply
- pharmaceutical hormones (birth control pills or HRT)
- impaired liver function (An unhealthy liver is unable to eliminate the majority of estrogen compounds from the body, so they are reabsorbed back into the bloodstream).

✓ To check the health of your liver, refer to the "Function of the Liver" in this manual.

Symptoms of estrogen dominance include:

- Acceleration of aging process
- Allergies
- Autoimmune disorders (strong correlation to BCP)
- Breast tenderness
- Breast, uterine, or ovarian cancer
- Decreased sex drive
- Depression
- Epilepsy
- Fatigue hypoglycemia
- Foggy thinking/ memory loss
- Gallbladder disease
- Hair loss
- Headaches
- Heavy menstrual bleeding and/or clots
- Increased blood clotting
- Infertility
- Insomnia
- Irritability
- Joint swelling
- Miscarriage
- PMS
- Premenopausal bone loss
- Thyroid dysfunction (mimicking hypothyroidism)
- Toxemia of pregnancy
- Uterine fibroids
- Water retention/bloating

Low estrogen is usually an issue at menopause or perimenopause. It affects you in body functions—hot flashes, night sweats, chills, heart palpitations, itching, and/or crawly skin—and mentally and emotionally—mood swings, irritability, anxiety, restlessness, panic attacks, nervousness, depression, forgetfulness, and/or mental distractions.

There are also physical signs:

- Insomnia
- Diminished sex drive

- Headaches or migraines more frequently
- Weight gain
- Frequent urination/incontinence
- Change of time between periods
- Hair loss
- Skin and vaginal dryness
- Fatigue
- Cold hands and feet—poor circulation
- Food allergies
- Leg cramps—bone pains, joint pain
- Growth of facial hair
- Nausea, gastric upset, bloating

Balance is *Essential*

Estrogen is not a singular hormone. The primary estrogens are:

1. Estrone—made in the liver. High levels are involved in cancer prevention.
2. Estriol—made mostly in the pituitary and adrenals.
3. Estradiol—made mostly in the pituitary and adrenals. High levels cause cancer (allow oxidation to take place in the cells).

Among these three of the basic estrogens, estradiol is most stimulating to the breast, and estriol is the least. Estradiol is 1,000 times more potent in its effects on breast tissue than estriol. Overexposure to estradiol increases one's risk of breast cancer; whereas, estriol is protective.

Note: BCP and traditional HRT use 100% Estradiol.

Role of Natural Progesterone:

1. Balances or opposes estrogen (prevents estrogen dominance)
2. Protects against cysts: breast, ovarian, thyroid
3. Protects against cancer
4. Normalizes blood clotting
5. Acts as a natural diuretic
6. Acts as a natural anti-depressant and relieves anxiety
7. Helps normalize blood sugar levels
8. Restores proper cell oxygen levels

9. Helps thyroid hormone function

10. Activates bone osteoclasts to increase new bone formation (reverses osteoporosis)

11. Helps use fat for energy

12. Beneficial anti-inflammatory effects (arthritis, MS, lupus)

13. Helps prevent hypertension

14. Prevents sinus, respiratory, and vaginal infections

15. Increases libido

16. Reduces hot flashes

17. Reduces risk of glaucoma

18. Reduces dryness and thinning of skin and hair loss

19. Essential for limbic brain health

The Progesterone Impostor

Both birth control pills and hormone replacement therapy contain Progestin. Side effects include an increased risk of blood clots, malignant mammary nodules, and sudden or partial loss of vision. It also may cause:

- Acne
- Alopecia (loss of hair)
- Anaphylactic allergic reactions
- Asthma
- Breast tenderness
- Depression
- Epilepsy
- Fluid retention
- Heart or kidney dysfunction
- Increased facial hair
- Insomnia Migraines
- Nausea
- Vaginal itch or infections

When Progestin was taken with estrogens, the following was observed:

- Cystitis
- Decrease in thyroid function
- Fatigue

- Headaches/dizziness
- Itching
- Joint pain
- Painful swellings of the legs
- PMS symptoms
- Rise in blood pressure
- Sudden onset of fever

Birth Control Pills

In reviewing women's health I came across the background of birth control pills. In 1951 Margaret Sanger is credited with convincing Gregory Pincus (who ultimately synthesized the first oral contraceptive) that his research in fertilization could be used to create an oral contraceptive. Available for the first time in the 1960's, oral contraceptives were truly a revolutionary medical option for women. "Women's maternal burden was lifted for the first time in history."[57] Writes author, Tori Hudson, N.D. in her book; *Women's Encyclopedia of Natural Medicine.*

To better understand this statement it is best to know who Margaret Sanger is. She was an official organizer for Planned Parenthood and author for a socialist newspaper. If children are a burden why does scripture tell us otherwise? It tells us they are a divine gift (Gen. 4:1, 33:5), they are promised as a reward of righteousness (Gen. 15:5, 22:17, Ex. 32:13; Lev. 26:9; Deut. 7:12-14; Ps. 45:16), come from God (Gen. 17:20; 29:31-35; 1 Sam. 1:19; Ps. 107:41), and are a blessing (Ps. 113:9; Prov. 10:1)

Innumerable happenings were taking place in the 60's as a cultural war without many Christians awareness. The Lone Star College – Kingwood web site[58] had this to say about the 60"s:

> The sixties were the age of youth, as 70 million children from the post-war baby boom became teenagers and young adults. The movement *away from the conservative* fifties continued and eventually resulted in revolutionary ways of thinking and real change in the cultural fabric of American life. No longer content to be images of the generation ahead of them, young people wanted change. The changes affected education, values, lifestyles, laws, and entertainment. Many of the revolutionary ideas which began in the sixties are continuing to evolve today.

> (Emphasis mine)

I am adding this personal rabbit chase in the middle of women's health for you to take a moment and think. Birth control pills change the chemistry of a woman's body. This can lead to problems later in life. When you look back and see how this paradigm switch came about during a revolution of challenging conservative beliefs, quite possibly these are areas we have eliminated God's control and added them to the list of "let man decide".

If this topic interests you then consider doing more research of your own. Natural pregnancy planning is vey common place in our society and there are various resources to choose from. In the Midwest, St. Louis, where I am from the local Catholic church teaches those who want to follow this method. It has worked very well for both of my girls – daughter and daughter in law. I am thankful they are looking out for their health and the health of their family.

Birth Control Leads to Abortions

How many of us take birth control pills without even thinking about what we are doing? We assume it is just to prevent a pregnancy but yet what the pills do is stop the baby from implanting into the uterus. Yes, it is already a baby at this point. Once America adopted acceptance of the BCP it was easier to go the next step and approve abortions. Since the day of Roe v. Wade the battle has been fought over human life in the home, courtroom and on the streets while the blood of babies continue to fill the troughs. We as Christians have been in the battle but not in the numbers of people that it should be.

Since the acceptance of the birth control pill the number of abortions has risen to where it is today with 1,200,000 babies killed every year under the pretense of 'convenience'. These babies are killed by dismembering their bodies, giving them a chemical bath to burn them alive, suctioning out their brain and other methods.

The medical side effects of such procedures lead to infertility, hemorrhage, and even death. This does not even take into account mentally what happens as the woman processes in her mind that she just killed an innocent baby because it interrupted her lifestyle.

Do I Need Hormone Replacement Therapy (HRT)?

After menopause, a woman should be able to produce all of the estrogen she needs *if* the following four glands are healthy: liver, ovaries, pituitary, and adrenals.

When a woman enters menopause, the ovaries do not completely stop producing estrogen, progesterone, or testerone. Usually the amount produced by the ovaries is about 40% of what they previously produced. God did not design your body to just stop. Your adrenal glands begin to make estrogen in the form of estrodiol and androgens, such as testerone, *but* only if the adrenal glands are working properly. The endocrine glands secrete hormones, the liver and the pituitary make hormones that are precursors to estrogens, but they have to be converted as you need them. This conversion process takes place in the body fat. If we are not making enough hormones, the body's survival mechanism to assist us is to make more fat to help out. This is why many women experience the "middle-age" spread. Your body will hold on to more fat if it needs to make more hormones.

Women with these problems should avoid HRT:

1. Cancer of the breast or uterus

2. Blood clots in the legs or lungs

3. High blood pressure

4. Active liver disease

5. Gallstones or gallbladder disease

6. Lupus, Crohns, rheumatoid arthritis, or any auto immune disease

Steps to Consider for Natural Hormone Balancing or Therapy
(This includes balancing hormones for PMS and perimenopause.)

Step 1: Diet

Eat...

Whole grains—including breads, cereals, pasta, pancakes, and waffles

Vegetables and fruits—increase fiber

Nuts, seeds—*flaxseed*

Soy products-organic only

Cold water fish—salmon, tuna, haddock

Water—drink ½ your body weight in ounces of water daily

Eliminate in your diet...

Alcohol	Refined sugar
Caffeine	Soft drinks
Saturated fats	Hydrogenated oils
Red meat	Homogenized dairy products

Step 2: Exercise—Nutrition's Twin

Exercise helps to reduce stress, along with getting your endocrine glands to be healthier. Reflect on positive thoughts, Bible verses, and prayers while exercising.

Step 3:   Nutritional Supplements

Consider these before going to a prescription:

1. Multi-vitamin
2. B-complex
3. Soy Protein—much research shows evidence of soy benefits
4. Vitamin C
5. Vitamin E
6. GLA—from the borage seed—three times stronger than primrose oil, major anti-inflammatory, major hormone builder.
7. EPA
8. Calcium
9. Magnesium
10. Flaxseed—grind your own—more nutrition

Step 4: Natural Hormone Therapy

1. Phytoestrogens: plant estrogens
2. Natural progesterone cream

Natural progesterone cream: usually during perimenopause the symptoms are due to estrogen dominance, too much estrogen, and not enough progesterone. Some women have had success with this type of natural hormone therapy.

> **WARNING:** This type of therapy can be tricky and hard to control the amounts applied and absorbed by the body, resulting in other problems with hormonal imbalances. Some women get messed up more with this cream.

Phytoestrogens are mild plant estrogen in certain plants, herbs, and seeds; are similar in chemical structure to estrogen; and have a hormone-like effect without the negative side-effects of synthetics hormones. Phytoestrogens are about 1,000th the strength of human estrogen (much weaker). Phytoestrogens respond to individual needs by stimulating estrogen production if levels are low and slowing down estrogen production if they are too high.

a. Lignin type in whole grains, vegetables, with highest concentration in oilseeds; grinding your own flaxseeds. This lignin is not present in flax oil.
b. Isoflavone type legumes with the highest concentration in protein are soybeans. There are hundreds of studies on the soy and hot flash connection.

 c. Herbs such as:

- Black Cohosh—helps with hot flashes, night sweats, calming effect on nervous system, helps regulate sleep patterns, vaginal dryness, fatigue
- Licorice root—promotes adrenal function
- Red Clover—helps detoxify the liver, enhances the immune system
- Don Quai—helps with hot flashes, vaginal dryness
- Panax Ginseng – reduces mental and physical fatigue, stress, ability to cope, vaginal changes

If you desire a supplement, the product I recommend is a combination of soy, black cohosh, flaxseed, dong quai, and licorice all in one capsule.

If You've Been taking HRT and Want to Stop All Hormones:

Don't stop cold turkey. Wean yourself gradually and slowly, giving your body time to adjust. Here's a sample weaning schedule:

Week 1: Skip Sunday's pill.
Week 2: Skip Sunday and Thursday.
Week 3: Skip Sunday, Tuesday, and Thursday.
Week 4: Skip Sunday, Tuesday, Thursday, and Saturday.
Week 5: Skip Sunday, Tuesday, Thursday, Friday, and Saturday.
Week 6: Get off hormones all together.

During and after this tapering off period, you will need to support your body by making sure you are getting enough plant hormones. Eat a wide variety of fruits and veggies, freshly ground flax seed, and soy. You'll also need a good multivitamin to help your adrenals and ovaries keep your hormones balanced. This guideline was suggested by Dr.Christiane Northrup in her book *The Wisdom of Menopause, Creating Physical and Emotional Health during the Change.*

Specific Symptoms and Recommended Supplement Guide:

In addition to a good multi-vitamin and grinding your own flax seed, add the following:

Hot flashes, night sweats, chills—soy protein, vitamin E, GLA

Anxiety, tension, panic attacks—B-Complex, calcium/magnesium, valerian

Vaginal Dryness—Vitamin E, GLA

Insomnia—Calcium/ Magnesium, valerian

Depression—B-complex, GLA, EPA, Soy protein

Memory, Concentration—lecithin, Ginkgo Biloba, B-Complex

Circulation—Vitamin E, Ginkgo Biloba, Co Enzyme Q10, EPA, Garlic, Lecithin, Vita C

Stress—B-Complex, Vitamin C, Soy protein

Fibrocystic Tendencies—Vitamin E, GLA

Fluid Retention—B- Complex, Soy protein, Alfalfa

Menstrual Cramps—Calcium magnesium, valerian

Headaches—Calcium magnesium, B-Complex, GLA, EPA

Diminished Sex Drive—Vitamin E, GLA

Dry Skin—EPA, GLA, Vitamin E, Carotenoids Complex

Heavy Periods or irregular periods—B-complex, GLA, EPA, Soy Protein

Anemia—Iron plus Vitamin C

Gas, Indigestion, bloating—Probiotic, chewable calcium/magnesium, peppermint and ginger in an herbal remedy

Acne—Probiotic, Zinc, Omega-3

Yeast and Bladder Infections—probiotic, garlic, Liver Detox, alfalfa

We can no longer afford to be weak or sick or tired or cranky or hormonally challenged. We all need to become our best selves, and we need to do it soon so as not to waste another minute settling for mediocrity. Each and every one of us is capable of feeling alive and vibrant.

HEALTHY HOME

I S YOUR HOME a haven? Since we spend a lot of time in our homes, it is time to search out any invaders robbing us of our health. Great health is achieved by addressing more than what we put in our bodies. We need to look at the environment in which our body lives. Omitting this step will leave us with possible toxin stowaways. Following are some easy steps to make your home your haven.

We are challenged by living in a world where the normal detoxification pathways lack normal stimulation and where abnormal exposures abound. This means as we try to over sterilize our homes of normal 'dirt' and allow in the toxic synthetic chemicals our immune system becomes overtaxed.

Getting Clean in Our Homes

Our Hands and Our Homes

God has given us skin as our first line of defense against infection. He made skin slightly acidic. It's called our "acid mantel." When we use a very alkaline, anti-bacterial, or deodorant soap, it destroys this acid mantel and germs are allowed in. Find soap that is pH-balanced. It will state this on the bottle, typically on the back label.

Recently we went on a cruise and they insisted everyone use their hand cleaner before going through the food line. I was prepared ahead of time and carried my own organic pH-balanced hand cleaner and revealed it to the ship personnel. They were kind enough to let us use our own cleaner.

The active ingredient in most antibacterial products is triclosan, an antibacterial agent that kills bacteria and inhibits bacterial growth. Triclosan is known to cause a range of health problems, from skin irritation to allergies. It stays in the environment a long time and can break down into dioxin in surface water. It also has been shown to kill human cells.[60] Since its introduction into consumer products in 1995, its use has spread rapidly.

Antibacterial ingredients are now in antibacterial soaps, laundry detergents, shampoos, toothpastes, body washes, dish soaps, and many household cleaning products. Consumers use these products because they have been marketed as an effective and necessary way to lower the risk of infection. However, many scientists fear the widespread use could lead to a strain of resistant bacteria, or "superbugs," and cause the ingredients to lose effectiveness for the times when they really are needed.

And now, the first major test in people's homes has found that using antibacterial products apparently offers little protection against the most common germs. In a recent study, people who used antibacterial soaps and cleansers developed coughs, runny noses, sore throats, fevers, vomiting, diarrhea, and other symptoms just as often, and sometimes more often, than people who used products that did not contain antibacterial ingredients.

The researchers pointed out that most of the symptoms experienced by the study participants are typically caused by viruses, which the antibacterial soaps don't protect against. And for the symptoms like vomiting and diarrhea, which may be caused by bacteria, the people who used regular soaps had no greater risk than those who used antibacterial products.[61]

So for healthy choices for you, your hands, and your home, look for organic pH-balanced cleaners. There are a few really good choices, so choose wisely. Look for a company that has been in the organic cleaner business for a long time and not just jumping on the green organic band wagon. If you need ideas, contact our office for suggestions and our favorite products.

Carcinogens to Avoid in Your Common Household Products

According to the book *The Safe Shoppers Bible, A Consumer's Guide to Nontoxic Household Products, Cosmetics, and Food* by David Steinman and Samuel Epstein, M.D., there are hundreds of common household products containing known carcinogens and/or neurotoxins. Carcinogens are chemicals that cause cancer. Neurotoxins are chemicals that adversely affect the nervous system, reducing emotional well being, mental alertness, coordination, and other functions associated with intelligence. I suggest you check this book out from the library and look up all the cleaners you are using in your home to see if they are known to include chemicals that cause cancer. You will be very surprised to find many of your favorite cleaners. In order to avoid this problem, it is recommended that you dispose of all cleaners that are not guaranteed to be organic for your health and green for the planet. It is worth the effort to find one of the few companies that really cares about your health and protecting it.

Begin by thinking of your home as a toxic waste dump. The average home today contains sixty-two toxic chemicals—more than a chemistry lab at the turn of the century. More than 72,000 synthetic chemicals have been produced since WWII.

Less than 2% of synthetic chemicals have been tested for toxicity, mutagenic, and carcinogenic effects or birth defects. And the majority of chemicals have never been tested for long-term effects. In the work place, Material Safety Data Sheets (MSDS) must accompany any product used. The work place and the outdoors are considered "legal environments," while the air in homes is not. So regulations for outdoor air pollution and toxins in the workplace are much stricter than in the home.

Health Effects of Chemical Exposure

Chemical exposure presents a real danger to you and your family's health and well-being. Even our beauty products are dangerous. The National Institute of Occupational Safety and Health has found more than 2,500 chemicals in cosmetics that are toxic, cause tumors, reproductive complications, biological mutations, and skin and eye irritations.

The health issues in this country have increased exponentially over the past few decades. Cancer rates have almost doubled since 1960. And as we have mentioned before, cancer is the number one cause of death for children. There has been a 26% increase in breast cancer since 1982. Breast cancer is the number one killer of women between the ages of thirty-five and fifty-four. Primary suspects are laundry detergents, household cleaners, and pesticides.

Since 1980, asthma has increased by 600%. The Canadian Lung Association and the Asthma Society of Canada identify common household cleaners and cosmetics as triggers. Also, ADD/ADHD is epidemic in schools today. Behavioral problems have long been linked to exposure to toxic chemicals and molds. Chemicals are attracted to and stored in fatty tissue. The brain is a prime target for these destructive organics because of its high fat content and very rich blood supply. Chemical and environmental sensitivities are known to cause all types of headaches.

Other diseases commonly related to chemical exposure include: fibromyalgia, chronic fatigue syndrome, arthritis, lupus, multiple sclerosis, circulatory disorders, Alzheimer's, Parkinson's disease, irritable bowel syndrome, depression, and hormonal problems.

Chemicals in Household Products

There are more than three million poisonings every year. Household cleaners are the number one cause of poisoning of children. The top three culprits, according to the Poison Control, are Household cleaners, bleach, and medications.

Formaldehyde is one of the largest indoor pollutants in our homes. Symptoms caused by formaldehyde are allergies, cancer, immune system failings, and asthma.

In brief, products containing formaldehyde include: antiperspirants, mouthwash, toothpaste, Tupperware, permanent press clothing, floor waxes, furniture polishes, baggies, coffee, wax paper, and paper money.

Phenols

Phenols are a major indoor pollutant. Phenols are absorbed by lungs and skin. Symptoms include caustic burns, kidney and liver damage, and hyperactivity. Products containing phenols include: acne medications, baking powder, computers, TV sets, mouthwash, sugar substitutes, and wallpaper.

Look for products that contain: no napthalene, no kerosene, no formaldehyde, no phenol, no creosol, no lye, no hydrochloric acid, no sulfuric acid, no petroleum distillates, no benzene, no ammonia, no Para dichlorobenzene, no sodium hydroxide, no butyl cello solve, no phosphoric acid, no chlorine, no phosphates, no nitrates, no borates, no animal testing, and are biodegradable.

Ways to Reduce Chemicals in Your Home and Keep Them from Entering Your Body

This list is not comprehensive, but it is a good start:

1. Do not destroy your "acid mantle" by using alkaline cleansers on your skin.
2. Do not smoke or stay in "smoky" or other harmful environments.
3. Drink only purified water.
4. Choose organically grown foods as much as possible. Many herbicides and pesticides contain chemicals that are hormone disrupters.
5. Always wash all fruits and vegetables well with a non-toxic cleanser.
6. Avoid plastic containers that contain organochlorines—PVCs: polyvinyl chloride. PVCs act as hormone disrupters.
7. Read product labels. Avoid preservatives, artificial colorings, and flavorings as much as possible.
8. Avoid heat-pressed oils, margarines, and fried foods, which contain trans-fatty acids.
9. Avoid sun protection products that contain harmful substances.
10. Avoid mosquito repellents that contain harmful substances.
11. Avoid all cosmetics, skin care, and personal care products that contain substances harmful to cellular tissue.
12. Avoid all household cleaners, laundry detergents, and dry cleaning solutions that contain substances harmful to cellular tissue. Avoid chlorine.
13. Use phosphate-free dishwasher detergent.

14. Store and microwave food in glass containers rather than plastics that contain PVCs. Remember, microwaved foods decrease white blood cells and affect the immune system.

15. Avoid lindane and synthetic pyrethroid-based head lice and scabies shampoo for humans and flea shampoo for pets.

16. Use natural lawn and garden maintenance methods.

17. If you golf, keep your hands, tees, and golf balls away from your mouth, since most golf courses are intensively sprayed.

18. Choose lead-free paint.

19. Avoid mercury amalgam dental fillings. Ask for porcelain, gold, or composite fillings.

20. Avoid chlorine as much as possible: Use an ozonator rather than chlorine in your swimming pool. Choose paper products bleached without the use of chlorine.

FLUORIDE

Fluoride is another confusing topic of our time. The effects in relation to our health of using fluoride in our drinking water and toothpaste are well documented on both sides by many researchers and scientists. Dentists are equally on opposing teams of this debate.

Whether or not to use fluoride is your decision. If you choose not to use fluoride for yourself and your family, your dentist can offer alternatives for teeth cleaning. There are many water purifiers that will remove this chemical from your drinking water also.

Fluoride comes from two different sources: industrial waste by-product or the natural element found in the earth. It is the processed waste by-product that is in question and the subject of this article. In our search to understand health, we need to continue to look back to the way our bodies were designed and the natural foods for best results.

Fluoride is a chemical that is added to our water supply "for our benefit." Typically, when man tries to improve on what was given to us naturally, those ideas causes me to take a second look. There are many reasons to purify our water due to the contamination of our water supply, but the addition of fluoride is for different reasons. This addition to our foods, water, toothpaste, and pharmaceuticals is reason to be educated and sometimes alarmed.

Dr. Paula Baile Hamilton, in her book *Toxic Overload*, discusses the health problems of fluoride:

Now scientist are linking fluoride to dental deformity and crippling bone disease. A recent report by the Greater Boston Physician for Social Responsibility reviews studies showing that fluoride interferes with brain functions in young animals and in children, reducing IQ. Some evidence suggests that fluoride products cause bone cancer in male rats and perhaps young men. Some European countries have recently banned most forms of fluoride products and are investigating bans of fluoride toothpaste. As of April 1997, toothpaste has been required to carry poison control information on the label as even a small amount, like a half a toothpaste tube full, can harm or kill a small child. Fluoride is also a hormone disrupter. Concentrations of fluoride are thought to be high enough in some toothpastes and mouthwashes to promote gingivitis as well as oral cancer.[61]

How much is too much?

As it turns out, too much toothpaste may not be good for your health. Concerned that too many young children were swallowing toothpaste, the Food and Drug Administration, beginning in April 1997, required the following warning to appear on tubes of fluoridated toothpaste: "Use only a pea sized amount and supervise child's brushing and rinsing (to minimize swallowing)." Parents also are warned to keep the toothpaste "out of the reach of children under 6," and to "seek professional help or contact a poison center immediately" if more than is used for brushing is accidentally swallowed.

The FDA's decision also was spurred by the growing number of cases of dental fluorosis—an unsightly and permanent discoloration of the teeth. The Wall Street Journal reports that twenty-two percent of American children now have the condition, which occurs in young children under six who have consumed too much fluoride.[62]

If your choice is to use toothpaste without fluoride, then there are several on the market. Your hunt will be rewarded.

FOOD ADDITIVES

Food additives are chemicals added to food to "improve" taste, texture, color, and shelf life. Additives came from the use of salt, smoke, spices, and sugars to preserve foods. Commercial food additives are regulated by governmental agencies. We will quickly look at some of these: sulfites, nitrites, salicylates, dyes, and MSG.

SULFITES: Sulfites are used to bleach and preserve food. They are often diagnosed as allergenic. Symptoms of sulfite allergies include flushing, dizziness, wheezing, or shortness of breath. Sulfite sprays are used on produce and on some salad bars. They are often found in wines, beers, and even in drugs. Sulfites are also used to keep the color of dried fruits. Recent governmental regulation has begun to limit their use. Purchasing organic fresh and dried fruits can help limit the intake of sulfites.

NITRATES: Nitrates, usually sodium salts, are frequently used in bacon and other processed meat (lunch meat, bologna, hotdogs). When they combine with some amino acids in the bowels, they can become carcinogenic. Vitamin C helps to inhibit this reaction. If you choose to eat foods with nitrates, be sure to take extra vitamin C supplementation or eat an orange.

SALICYLATES: The grandfather of salicylates is aspirin. Salicylates can also be found in foods. It can trigger asthma and has been implicated in deaths due to respiratory failure. Dr. Feingold has done extensive research in the areas of salicylates, allergies, and children's behavior problems. You can contact the Feingold Organization at 703-768-3287 for more information on salicylates and children.

FOOD DYES: Dyes have often been associated with allergic reactions and behavioral problems in children. Food dyes are used in many commercial food products. Any item with a number (i.e., #5) in an ingredient list is an example of a food dye. Food coloring used at home is another example. Yellow food coloring has been associated with hives. It is often found in commercial pasta and cookies. Symptoms occurring within ninety minutes of ingesting can include asthma, hives, swelling, headaches, and behavior changes. Safe alternatives are plant-based colors, such as beet juice.

MONOSODIUM GLUTAMATE (MSG): MSG continues to be a controversial additive. MSG is a food enhancer. It can cause headaches, bloating, and other side effects. Severe sensitivities to MSG can cause shock. Read more about this under the title "MSG" in this manual.

PESTICIDES

According to the Code of Federal Regulations 162.10, it is illegal to claim that a pesticide is safe, even if the label contains a qualifying phrase such as "when used as directed." Children who live in homes in which household and garden pesticides are used have a greater chance of developing illness. In a 1983 San Francisco survey, DDT was found to be the most common pesticide residue found on fresh produce. (Although DDT has been banned since 1972, over forty years later it is still showing up in crops and cord blood of new born babies).

Farmers have added pesticides to reduce insect damage and increase crop production. Yet, interestingly enough, while the use of agricultural pesticides has increased tenfold in the last thirty years, crop losses due to insects have doubled. It is also interesting to note that a pesticide that has been previously banned for use in this country can still be used if the EPA grants an emergency waiver.

Pesticides can remain active for days, weeks, and even years. A common misconception about pesticide applications is that the pesticide is no longer harmful after it has "dried." The fact is that some pesticides have a half life of fifty to seventy-five years (DDT, for example). Of the 35,000 pesticides used in the U S, only 10% have been tested. When US-outlawed pesticides are exported, they are used on the foods we import. Typically, imported foods tend to have more pesticides.

When you simply wash produce (grown with pesticides), nothing happens. Most pesticides are formulated to be water-resistant. Wash all produce with an organic vegetable wash and a natural brush to remove as much of the pesticide as possible.

Spraying lawns and gardens for bugs can cause tremendous side effects. Since pesticides are designed to impact the "pest's" nervous systems, it will also affect yours.

So, what are the *solutions* to these issues? Organic food is grown without the use of chemicals. In California, "organic" is defined as food that is "produced, harvested, distributed, stored, processed and packaged without the application of synthetically compounded fertilizers, pesticides or growth regulators." This is different from "pesticide-free" labels. "Pesticide-free" indicates that a random inspection of the food was done at the docks and no pesticides were detected at that time. However, half of pesticides applied cannot be detected with these routine tests.

Homemade Remedies for Pests

- **Insects:** Diluted cayenne pepper, chili pepper, paprika, or dried peppermint can be used to repel most insects.
- **Moles:** Dump several scoops of used cat litter into the mole's tunnel; moles find it offensive and will leave. Don't, however, spread cat litter near a food garden because it can carry infections harmful to humans.
- **Mice:** Inexpensive snap traps from the hardware store are quite effective when deployed in large numbers. Set baited traps at two-foot intervals along the base of walls where mice run. To kill both young and old mice, set traps out twice: once to trap the adults, and then two weeks later to trap maturing young. Bait traps with peanut butter or with a small cotton ball. Mice pull at the cotton when they are collecting nesting material and so trigger the trap; unlike food baits, cotton doesn't spoil in hot weather. To avoid leaving a telltale human odor, always wear gloves when handling traps.
- **Aphids, mealy bugs, mites, scales, and thrips:** Make a soap spray. Mix one tablespoon dishwashing soap in one gallon of water. Test the spray on a few leaves of the affected plant; if no damage results, spray the whole plant.
  You also can make an ammonia spray by mixing one part household ammonia with seven parts water. Or make an oil spray by stirring one tablespoon of liquid dishwashing soap into one cup of vegetable oil (peanut, safflower, corn, soybean, or sunflower). Mix 1 to 2 teaspoons of the soap and oil blend with one cup water, and apply to affected plants.
- **Ants:** To keep a pet's food from attracting ants, set the food dish in a pie pan filled with soapy water.
  You can use mint or lavender to repel ants. Spray ants with clove oil diluted in arm soapy water.
  To destroy invading ant colonies, mix three cups of water with one cup of sugar and four teaspoons of boric acid. Loosely pack several small screw top jars half full with

cotton balls, saturated with the mixture. Pierce jar lids with two to three small holes (large enough to admit ants) and screw back onto jars. Place jars in areas where ants are active but out of the reach of children and pets.

- **Rabbits:** Plant French marigolds amid rabbit delicacies, such as lettuce and carrots, in the vegetable garden. The marigolds' strong odor repels rabbits. Sprinkle ground pepper around plants to repel rabbits—renew after every rain.
- **Roaches:** Use garlic and bay leaves to help keep roaches away.

FOODS WITH HIGHEST AND LOWEST PESTICIDE RESIDUE

What fruits and veggies are best and worst when it comes to pesticide residues? Here is a summary of pesticides-in-food data. The main source is research conducted by the Environmental Working Group (EWG), but these results have been augmented with additional information from analyses performed by Charles M. Benbrook, Ph.D., an agricultural specialist, and by Consumers Union. There are four categories, from worst to best. Updated 2014.

Eating fruits and vegetables with pesticides is still a better choice than not eating these raw foods at all. This range from Avoid to Best of the Bunch gives a view of how to shop in

Avoid unless Organic:	*Use Caution:*	*Better…Not Perfect*	*Best of the Bunch*
Apples	Blueberries	Tangerines	Mushrooms
Strawberries	Lettuce	Summer Squash	Sweet potatoes
Grapes	Snap Peas - imported	Broccoli	Cantaloupe
Celery	Kale/ collard greens	Winter squash	Grapefruit
Peaches	Cherries	Green onions	Kiwi
Spinach	Nectarines - domestic	Snap peas – domestic	Eggplant
Sweet Bell Peppers	Pears	Oranges	Asparagus
Nectarines - imported	Plums	Tomatoes	Mangoes
Cucumbers	Raspberries	Honeydew melon	Papayas
Potatoes	Blueberries – imported	Cauliflower	Sweet peas frozen
Cherry Tomatoes	Carrots	Bananas	Cabbage
Hot peppers	Green beans	Watermelon	Avocados
			Pineapples
			Onions
			Sweet corn (possible GMO)

the store. When choosing foods from the avoid list, this is an opportunity to try organic. Even the foods listed in the Best of the Bunch column were not always found to be pesticide-free, but they were consistently low in pesticide residues and are your best choices for non-organic foods. An EWG simulation showed that people can lower their pesticide exposure 90% by avoiding the most contaminated fruits and vegetables.

MSG—MONOSODIUM GLUTAMATE

What Is It?

MSG is a food additive that enhances flavors in food while having virtually no flavor of its own. How it adds flavor to other foods is not fully understood, but people do experience a more intense flavor from foods containing MSG. It is a simple, inexpensive way for the food industry to enhance flavors, mask unwanted tastes, and hide undesirable flavors in foods.

MSG is the sodium salt of the amino acid glutamic acid and a form of glutamate. It is sold as a fine white crystalline substance, similar in appearance to salt or sugar.

Glutamate is found in many living things. It occurs naturally in our bodies and in protein-containing foods, such as cheese, milk, meat, peas, tomatoes, and mushrooms. This natural form found in food is not the problem; however, it is the pure synthetic crystalline MSG that creates havoc. In other words, it is the chemical substance that man has created that is causing us problems.

Names of MSG (this is just an example; there are now over 40 names for MSG)

- Autolyzed yeast
- Calcium caseinate
- Hydrolyzed milk protein
- Kombu
- Sodium caseinate
- Yeast extract
- Broth*
- Casein
- Hydrolyzed protein
- Natural flavor
- Stock

*"Natural flavors," "stock," and "broth" can mean MSG is an added ingredient, or it can mean many other ingredients, but it is a wording that the manufacturers are allowed to use to hide their trade secrets. You as the consumer have no way of knowing if MSG is in the product.

Health Problems with MSG

Some people have a reaction to eating MSG that can happen in one hour or up to forty-eight hours later. Some symptoms of a reaction to MSG are:

Other health problems that can result:

- Damage to the Central Nervous System
- Endocrine organ disorders

- Anxiety
- Chest pain
- Diarrhea
- Dizziness
- Excessive sweating
- Facial pressure
- Hyperactivity
- Migraine headaches
- Mood changes
- Nausea

- Panic attacks
- Rapid heart beat
- Skin flushing
- Sleep problems
- Burning sensation in the back of the neck, forearms, and chest
- Numbness in the back of the neck radiating to the arms and back
- Tingling, warmth, and weakness in the face

- Cardiac arrest
- Alzheimer's disease
- ALS or Lou Gehrig's disease
- Obesity—leading to type 2 diabetes

Labeling

The government has designated MSG as a generally regarded as safe (GRAS) ingredient. There is much controversy to this labeling, and many organizations are fighting to ban the use of this ingredient. Many companies are adapting and placing "No MSG" on their labels, but the ingredients may still list autolyzed yeast or hydrolyzed protein, which are forms of MSG. The manufacturers claim MSG is a naturally-occurring ingredient, but there are lots of naturally-occurring substances that are undesirable for your body. The answer here is that we don't need the synthetic MSG added to our foods.

Further Study

The MSG manufacturers themselves admit that it addicts people to their products. It makes people choose their product over others, and makes people eat more of it than they would if MSG wasn't added. Not only is MSG scientifically proven to cause obesity, but also it is an addictive substance!

With one exception, aspartame and processed free glutamic acid (MSG) cause identical adverse reactions in people who are sensitive to them. In addition, the free glutamic acid found in MSG and the free aspartic acid found in aspartame both have been shown to kill brain cells and cause subsequent endocrine disorders in laboratory animals.

There are many web sites, books, and studies about the effects of MSG on our health. Since the problem comes for the synthetic form of MSG and not the naturally derived forms it is best to eliminate this ingredient whenever possible to prevent health problems.

Information gathered for this article comes from many resources but primarily www.truthinlableing.org.

XENOBIOTICS

<u>Definition</u>: Foreign substances originating outside the body that have "hormone-like" and "estrogen-like" activity in the body.

Result: A profound impact on hormone balance.
Xenobiotics: A" generic" reference to substances with a hormone-like effects on the body.
Xenoestrogens: Xenobiotics that have an estrogenic effect on the body.

What do Hormones do?
They are chemical messengers produced by the endocrine glands that:

- Inform cells about how and when to grow.
- Regulate many biological processes.
- Guide the development of sexual organs, nervous and immune systems, organs and tissues (such as the liver), blood, kidneys, muscles, and brain.

Hormone-Related Problems caused by Xenobiotics:

- Declining sperm count
- Climbing rates of cancer of the reproductive tract, including breast, testicular, and prostate
- Infertility
- Feminization of males
- Masculinization of females
- Increasing incidence of hyperactivity and learning disorders

The developing fetus and young children are thought to be at the greatest risk because of the hormonal activity that occurs in the development of their immune, nervous, and reproductive systems.

How to Avoid Xenobiotics

- Choose non-toxic xenobiotic-free cleaners.
- Avoid chlorine.
- Choose non-toxic, xenobiotic-free personal care products, such as toothpaste, shampoo, cream rinse, hairspray, etc.
- Use only plastic containers that contain "No PVCs."
- Purchase organically grown foods as much as possible.
- Wash fruits and veggies in an organic cleaner to cut the petro-based sprays.
- Use natural lawn and garden care methods.
- Eat ocean fish as compared to lake fish.
- Drink only filtered water.
- Don't smoke, and stay away from smoky areas.
- Avoid all synthetic vitamins—even many natural vitamins contain xenobiotics as solvents.
- Detoxify xenobiotics from your system on a daily basis.

Common Xenobiotics found in Cleaners

Xenobiotic	Used In
Ammonia	cleaners, degreasing agents
Cresol	disinfectants
Nonylphenol	liquid laundry
Ethoxylates	detergents, soaps
Phenols	laundry detergents, disinfectants
Formaldehyde	disinfectants, germicides
Sodium Hypochlorite	bleaching agents
Sodium Hydroxide	drain cleaners, oven cleaners
Oxalic Acid	furniture polish
Trichloroethylene	solvents and degreasers
Phenyl phenol	disinfectant fungicides
Chlorine	disinfectants and brighteners
Dioxins	disinfectants

PLASTICS: IT'S ALL IN THE NUMBERS! OR IS IT?

Did you know? More than one hundred pesticide ingredients are suspected to cause birth defects, cancer and gene mutations. More than 1 million children are exposed to unsafe levels of pesticides in their food.

~Paula Baillie-Hamilton, M.D., Ph. D. author of *Toxic Overload*.

Before any food reaches your mouth, there are many ways in which chemicals can still sneak into it. Plastic or metal packaging, cooking containers, utensils, and food coverings can all contaminate food with toxic chemicals. In fact, the chemicals in plastic are highly fat soluble; so many fatty foods placed in direct contact with a plastic act like blotting paper and absorb the toxins directly from the plastic.

Most of the foods we purchase come in one of three different containers: plastic, glass, or paper. Of the three, plastic is the most widely used and convenient. Unfortunately, the health problems related to plastic vary from hormone disruption to thyroid damage. The numbers of studies that are available to the public are numerous. But the bottom line is that you must understand the numbers.

The Society of the Plastics Industry created an easy to understand plastic recycling code that immediately identifies the type of plastic you're bringing into your life. Let's review them and see how they should be used and the possibilities of health problems associated with each number.

- #1 PET or PETE (polyethylene terephthalate) is used to make most clear soda and water bottles. It can be recycled into carpet fibers and rope.
- #2 HDPE (high density polyethylene) appears in such items as "cloudy" milk jugs, water bottles, and detergent bottles. It is recycled as trash cans, traffic cones, and more detergent bottles.
- #3 PVC or V (polyvinyl chloride) is used for beach balls and toys, cooking oil bottles, fast-food serving containers, pacifiers, raincoats and boots, some soft bottles, shampoo bottles, and plastic trays in boxed cookies.
- #4 LDPE (low-density polyethylene) is used to make shrink wrap, food storage bags, plastic grocery bags, and margarine tub tops. It recycles as new grocery bags.
- #5 PP (polypropylene) goes into bottle caps, rigid containers such as yogurt cups and syrup bottles, and plastic straws. It can be recycled into car battery cases and plastic lumber.
- #6 PS (polystyrene) is found in disposable coffee cups (Styrofoam), packaging peanuts, some plastic cutlery and egg cartons, and clam-style food containers. It recycles as flower pots and plastic lumber.
- #7 Other (generally polycarbonate) Plastics in this category appear as microwaveable

dishes, five-gallon water bottles, baby bottles, eating utensils, lining for metal cans, dental sealants, and catsup squeeze bottles.

In order for things to be safe for your family, glass is always the best choice. The numbers change from year to year, so make wise choices.

- *Better choices* are #5, #4, and #2. #1 and #2 are the most commonly recycled.
- *Worst Choices* #3, #6, and #7 should be avoided whenever possible.

These choices are one viewpoint. Other people feel that different numbers are best. That is why I choose glass whenever possible.

Let's take a closer look:
- #3: Commonly used to package foods and liquids, toys, teethers, plumbing and building supplies. This chlorinated form of plastic contains numerous toxic chemicals called adipates and phthalates (plasticizers), which are used to soften brittle PVC into a more flexible form. The WHO International Agency for Research on Cancer has recognized the chemical used to make this plastic, vinyl chloride, as a known human carcinogen. The European Union has banned the use in children's toys. Traces of these chemicals can leach out when it comes in contact with food.
- Earl Gray, Ph. D., EPA, specialist in hormone-altering chemicals says there is no doubt that phthalates block male hormones and result in reproductive feminization in lab animals. Recent studies found that pregnant women using beauty products containing phthalates had male babies with smaller genitals.
- #6: Styrene is on the toxins that the EPA monitors in our drinking water. Some compounds leaching from the Styrofoam food containers interfere with hormone functions. Is also has been identified as a human carcinogen.
- #7: This product is a known hormone disrupter that releases into food and liquid and acts much like estrogen. Research in Environmental Health Perspectives finds it can increase body weight of lab animals' offspring as well as impact hormone levels.
- A more recent study suggests that even low-level exposure results in insulin resistance, which can eventually lead to inflammation and heart disease. The EPA researchers conclude that exposure to BPA (found in this plastic) raises the risk of high blood pressure, high cholesterol, and type 2 diabetes—now reaching epidemic proportions in this country.

Simple Steps to Better Health Regarding Plastics

It can be overwhelming when we consider the many uses that plastic is used for in our homes. Let's start with a few simple changes, and over time, switching to alternatives from plastic packaging will be an easy choice.

1. Select biodegradable packaging whenever possible, such as waxed paper rather than plastic.

2. Look for eggs packed in cardboard.

3. Wash out glass jars and containers, and reuse them to store foods and liquids.

4. Buy in bulk, and transfer your purchases to your own glass containers when you get home.

5. Scrape off the top layer of fatty foods (such as cheese and meat) that has come into contact with plastic wrap and store the food in glass and ceramic.

6. Never use plastic wrap when heating foods, instead, heat foods and drinks in ovenproof glass or ceramic.

7. If something tastes like plastic, don't drink or eat it. Chances are plastic has leached into the food or drink.

8. Don't rewash and reuse plastic bottles, as this can accelerate the breakdown of materials. Look for baby bottles made of glass or opaque, pastel-colored #4 or #5 plastic.

CONCLUSION

Glorify God in Your Body

MAN'S OPTION TO choose whether or not he will care for his body and spirit is shown in the last sentence of 1 Corinthians 6:20: "Therefore glorify God in your body and in your spirit, which are God's." God has given man a free will to choose for himself. But he has also given man rules by which to live. God knows that for man to be truly happy, he must obey and live his life according to God's directives.

Two good examples of God's directives that lead us to happiness are: "You shall love the Lord you God with all your heart, and with all your soul, and with all your mind, and with all your strength" (Mark 12:30, RSV); and learn to "love your neighbor as yourself" (v.33, RSV). Many Christians who stray from his direction experience unhappiness from choosing the wrong lifestyle. We all stray, and many of us are still learning to put God first in our life.

In this verse God provides another rule that will contribute to our happiness. He is directing us to glorify him in our bodies to the best of our ability, and to condition our bodies to their optimum physical capability. If we obey this directive, we will more likely remain healthy throughout our lives. Good health will enhance our service for him, and we can serve more effectively without stress and fatigue.

Many Christians choose to neglect this directive. They let false pleasures dominate their bodies. Many overeat, eat foods without nutritional value, drink alcohol, smoke tobacco, worry unnecessarily, and avoid every opportunity to exercise. This lifestyle is prevalent among Christians of all denominations. This includes many Christians who are obedient to God's spiritual laws; they attend church regularly, tithe, and serve others with compassion and concern, but do not glorify God in their bodies. This lack of obedience to God's command is sin. I feel it is sin to neglect the physical needs of God's temple.

Sins against the body are costly. Our bodies deteriorate from heart disease, high blood pressure, diabetes, and lower back disorders, which, in many instances, can be prevented by proper nutrition and exercise. Christian, you have a choice. You can neglect your body's physical needs, which lead to poor health, or glorify God in your body, which often leads to good health. Your witness to the world and your wellbeing depend on the choices you make.

In closing, our prayer to you is that you will be able to make healthy choices to benefit your body. From there you will have the vitality and energy to either travel the world or go across the street to share the good news of Jesus with your neighbor. This is our prayer for you:

Beloved, I pray that in all respects you may prosper and be in good health, just as your soul prospers. For I was very glad when brethren came and bore witness to your truth, that is, how you are walking in truth. I have no greater joy than this, to hear of my children walking in the truth.

3 John 2–4

RESOURCES

Cooking Healthy

MANY OPINIONS ABOUND when it comes to healthy cookware. Waterless stainless steel is by far still the best choice. I have been using my set for over twenty-five years and it still cooks as if it were brand new. Royal Prestige is a company you can trust. The investment is worth the health and taste benefits. Here is their contact info to get more information.

Royal Prestige Cookware

Royal Prestige – R.P. Spectrum, Inc.
Web site: www.rphealthspectrum.com
Email: info@rphealthspectrum.com
Phone: 1- 888-80BRIDE

BAKING HEALTHY

Getting Started Making Bread

What you need to get started with mixer mixing:

- BOSCH MIXER: This high quality mixer will make all recipes fun and quick. If you have a Kitchen Aid, only make two loaves at a time and let the machine rest, it is not designed to handle the five-loaf recipe in the *Healthy Treasures* cookbook.
- NUTRIMILL: A high-quality electric grain mill such as the Nutrimill (I like this better than the Wondermill.)

- BREAD PANS: Four of the eight-inch waffle weave or stainless steel loaf pans (You can buy various sizes.)
- YEAST: The vacuum packed SAF yeast is less expensive than the packets or bottles in your local grocery store. The vacuum packed packages can be found online, (see resource section) at some Mediterranean stores, or at some health food stores.
- REAL SALT: this is the least processed brand of sea salt. There are lots of sea salt varieties in all stores, so be choosy and choose the highest quality. You will find many trace minerals in this brand that can be lost from the sea salt during processing.
- DOUGH SCRAPER: One dough scraper – makes it fun and easy to work with dough
- BREAD BAGS: Heavy duty bread bags (washable, reusable)
- WHEAT
  - Hard Red
  - Hard White
  - Soft White – pastry
- Other options include Spelt, Kamut, etc.

What you need to get started with a bread machine:

- A high-quality electric grain mill such as the Nutrimill
- A good quality bread machine such as the Zojuirishi (programmable horizontal loaf)
- Package of yeast
- Real Salt
- Heavy duty bread bags
- Wheat:
  - Hard Red
  - Hard White
  - Soft White
- Other options include spelt, kamut, etc.

What you need to get started with hand kneading:

- A high-quality electric grain mill such as the Nutrimill
- Package of yeast
- Real Salt
- Heavy duty bread bags
- One dough scraper
- Wheat:
  - Hard Red

- Hard White
- Soft White
- Other options include spelt, kamut, etc.

Baking Equipment and Supplies

For most of your baking needs check out our website: www.designedhealthyliving.com . Or call 804-798-6565 for personal assistance and specials.

Grains

When buying grains it is best to buy your first bag of grain in a bucket and also purchase a Gamma Lid. This saves your fingers each time you go to open the bucket. The purchases after that do not need to be in the bucket, since the bucket lasts a lifetime.

Nutrimill

The Nutrimill, makes grain, beans, legumes and corn into a fine flour that makes wonderful bread and tasty cakes. This one unit is convenient to use and worth every dollar in the convenience of having a grain mill in your very own home.

BOSCH Universal Plus, mixer makes it easy to make five loaves of bread at one time. Check it out at Country Baker or call our office to see if we have them in stock to send you one.

Features:
- 800 Watts
- 6 ½ quart bowl
- 4 speed settings + momentary switch
- Cord storage
- Suction feet for a secure standing
- Wide range of optional accessories
- Overload and start motor protection
- Easy to clean
- 3-year motor/transmission warranty

Selling Features:
- BOSCH quality—average lifetime for mixers is 17 years
- The most powerful motor in its class
- Unique and modern design

- Large mixing bowls handle up to 15 lbs of dough
- Ergonomic and easy handling with rim at top of bowl
- Works perfectly whether small or large quantities (as little as one egg white)
- Endless possibilities with optional accessories (listed on the back)
- Removable drive shaft is easy to clean
- Whisk holder is dishwasher safe
- Splash ring allows for easy adding of ingredients
- Sealed oil transmission more than doubles the lifetime of the transmission
- Dough hook is designed to replicate hand kneading

Benefits

- BOSCH quality—higher average lifetime for mixers in its class
- High customer satisfaction
- BOSCH has sold this series of mixer since the 1950's.
- Long term, proven quality and performance
- Dough hook: designed to simulate hand kneading process
- Dough hook creates 100% gluten development in minimal time.

Attachments: Blender, cookie paddles, slicer/shredder, plus many more attachments to make cooking fun.

RPM blender

Features:

- 900 Watts
- 7 Cup blender capacity
- Commercial designed stainless steel blades and assembly
- Heavy duty polycarbonate pitcher and smoothie stick
- Brushed metal housing block base
- On/off toggle switch
- Unique tachometer shows operating speed
- 6-year warranty

Selling Features:

- Unique and modern design
- Chops ice to snow

- Variable speed control between 500 and 20,000 RPMs
- Opening in lid allows for easy adding of ingredients
- Blender jar is dishwasher safe (blades are not)
- Easy to clean

Benefits:

- Voted Favorite blender by *Men's Journal* Magazine
- This blender is a must for every kitchen.
- Best performance for an affordable price
- Liquefies in a matter of seconds
- Harvest time – use your blender for delicious homemade soups
- Prepare quick and easy healthy food for your baby.
- The perfect blender to compliment any party—cocktails, dips, and deserts
- This L'Equip model is manufactured of the highest quality. It is a really user-friendly health appliance that not only performs well, but has a unique design to complement any kitchen.

GROCERY SHOPPING GUIDE

Consider yourself on a treasure hunt as you discover new foods to wow your taste buds. As you begin looking for health building foods, it is important to look at the perimeter of the grocery store. That is typically where "live" foods are located. Try to ensure the majority of your diet consists of these foods, foods that may rot fairly quickly. Many bakery goods have lasted for up to two years! It is hard to imagine the nutritional value in such a food.

Your kids' eating choices directly reflect your own, for the most part. It is important to instill healthy eating habits at an early age to ensure long-term health. Make it fun when possible, but be firm. You may even need to be firm with yourself. This is one of those "battles" that is worth it in the long run.

A Grocery Shopping Guide is available for printing at the Designed Healthy Living Web site. This useful tool takes the guesswork out of shopping.

Resources and Suppliers

Consultations

Designed Healthy Living has a network of professional consultants who are trained in the biblical design of our health. Readers who have purchased this book along with the

Treasures of Healthy Living Bible Study are given a free 30-minute consultation for answers to food and supplement questions. To schedule an appointment call 1-804-798-6565 or email: yourfriends@designedhealthyliving.com.

Cookbooks

Healthy Treasures Cookbook: This is a collection of great tasting, healthy recipes featuring ingredients to build health. You will be surprised and delighted that you can please your family with tasteful dishes while contributing to their well being. This cookbook is available through the Designed Healthy Living Web site, Barnes and Noble, and Amazon Web sites. Or by emailing yourfriends@designedhealthyliving.com.

Cookware

Royal Prestige – R.P. Spectrum, Inc. Email: info@rphealthspectrum.com; 1- 888-80BRIDE, www.rphealthspectrum.com

Food Co-op

www.quailcovefarms.com
www.localharvest.com
www.breadbeckers.com

Supplements and Organic Cleaners

Because of FDA guidelines we are not allowed to share the brand names of supplements we recommend. In Value Your Vitamins you can read *Consumer Checklist for High-Quality Vitamin Supplements.* These guidelines will direct you to only the top quality companies. It is worth your time to research this topic. For personal recommendations please contact our office (yourfriends@designedhealthyliving.com or 804-798-6565).

READING AND RESEARCH

Web sites:

Cancer Prevention Coalition, www.preventcancer.com

The National Institute of Occupational Safety and Health Web site

Environmental Working Group www.ewg.org

> For skin care products reports: www.ewg.org/reports/skindeep
>
> Local co-ops, restaurants, farmers markets, etc. www.localharvest.org

Reading Materials

Believing God by Beth Moore: As you begin a new eating plan, this book will help you learn how to believe in God during the process of change.

Digestive Wellness by Elizabeth Lipski

Dying to Look Good: by Christine Hoza Farlow

Fast Food Nation by Eric Schlosser: This is an interesting look at the food being served at the fast food restaurants. Do not read if you want to continue eating out and ignoring the facts.

Fats That Heal, Fats That Kill by Udo Erasmus: This book helps to understand the different fats in our foods and how they relate to our bodies.

Food Additives by Christine Hoza Farlow

Fresh Wind, Fresh Fire by Jim Cymbala—Prayer is vital to everything we are doing in our lives which includes our health. This book gives a fresh look our prayer life.

Getting a Handle on Your Emotions by Adrian Rogers, Love Worth Finding Ministries

How to Raise a Healthy Child in Spite of Your Doctor by Robert S. Mendelssohn, M.D. – This pediatrician gives sound advice to help you keep your children healthy and if they get sick he instructs you how to heal them at home to avoid going to the doctor. Very common sense advice on fevers, earaches, sore throats, etc.

Is This Your Child? By Doris Rapp, M.D.

Is This Your Child's World? By Doris Rapp, M.D.

Leaky Gut Syndrome by Elizabeth Lipski

More than Enough by Dave Ramsey: Financially free allows us as much freedom as being healthy. Debt free contributes to our health. This is a must read.

Planning, Planting and Harvesting Your Herb Garden by Marianne Mittwede Ritchie – This book must be ordered by mail: Po Box 852, Midlothian Virginia 23113, email: tym2plnt@hotmail.com or phone: 804-594-0667

Praying God's Word by Beth Moore

Prescription for Nutritional Healing by Balch

Prescription for Dietary Wellness by Balch

The Safe Shopper's Bible by Macmillan, 1995 ed.

The Vaccine Guide, Risks and Benefits for Children and Adults by R. Neustaedter: This book gives a balanced approach to vaccines—which ones are necessary, which ones to avoid, and what the best timeframe is for receiving vaccines.

The Wisdom of Menopause by Christiane Northrup, M.D. This book gives some great understanding about all the cycles of a women's life. Some of her views may conflict with Christianity but her facts about our health are very beneficial.

The Yeast Connection by William G. Crooke

Toxic Overload by Paula Baillie-Hamilton, M.D., Ph.D. This author has completed many studies on the chemical calorie and the effects of toxins in our bodies.

You Can Prevent Breast Cancer by Harry Diamond. This book is beneficial in understanding how fasting can relieve your body of toxins and specifically the toxins that build up in breast tissue.

Background Sources

Besides the numerous textbooks on nutrition and health sciences the list below represents the principal works referred to in the text, as well as others that supplied facts and influenced this writing. Web site URLs are current as of March 2014.

American Journal of Clinical Nutrition, April, 2002.

Annie Graves, *Know Your Plastics* by Annie Graves, Taste for Life, January, 2007.

Bernard Ward, *Healing Foods from the Bible* (New York: Globe Communications, 1994).

Bonnie Morrell, *Healthy Living* (Atlanta, Georgia, Wellness Seminar, 2002)

Christiane Northrup, M.D., *The Wisdom of Menopause*, (New York, Bantam Books, 2001)

Christine Gaber, RHN and Charlene Day, RDC , *Why Do I Feel This Way?* (Ontario, Canada, Health Thru Knowledge Pub, 2008).

Donna G. Spann, *Grains of truth, Using Whole Grains the Easy Way* (Lorton, Virginia, Today's Family Matters Pub, 2005).

Doris Rapp, M.D., *Is This Your Child?* (New York, Bantam Books, 1996).

Doris Rapp, M.D., *Is This Your Child's World* (New York, Bantam Books, 1993).

Dr. Bruce Miller, *Eating Right for a Bad Gut* (Texas, Miller Enterprises, 2003).

Dr. Bruce Miller, *Prostate Health, What's New*, publication volume 26, issue 2.

Dr. Richard Brouse, *Practical Nutrition*, Lecture Seminar, 2007.

Earl Mindell, Ph.D., *Herb Bible* (New York, Simon and Schuster, 1992.)

Elizabeth Lipski, M.S., CCN, D*igestive Wellness* and *Leaky Gut Syndrome* (Los Angeles, Keats Publishing, 1996).

Gemma Gorham, MPH, *Natural Approaches to Prostate Health*, seminar literature.

John Lee, M.D., *What Your Doctor May Not Tell you about Menopause* (New York, Warner Books, 1996).

John Lust, N.D., D.B.M., *The Herb Book*, Bantam Books, 1974.

Marion Nestle, *What to Eat* (New York, North Point Press, 2006)

Martha Wilmore, CDC, *Male Concerns*, Seminar literature.

Martha Wilmore, CDC, Nutritionists in Canada, Seminar Literature.

Pastor Jeff Brauer, Winn's Baptist Church, Virginia, sermon notes.

Paula Baillie-Hamilton, *Toxic Overload* (New York, Penguin Press, 2005).

Phyllis Balch*, Prescription for Dietary Wellness* (New York, Avery Pub., 2003).

Plasticizers Go from Breast Milk to Baby, Environmental Science and Technology, 7/12/06.

Richard Couey, Ph.D., *Nutrition for God's Temple* (Nashville, Life-way Press, 1994).

Rusty Ost, RPH, Phyto-Bytes, Co Q Heart, 2007.

Samuel S. Epstein, M.D., and David Steinman, *The Safe Shopper's Bible* (New Jersey, Wiley Publishing, 1995).

Sloan Barnett, *Green Goes With Everything, Simple Steps to a Healthier Life and a Cleaner Planet* (New York, Atria Books, 2008).

Steve Meyerowitz, *Water, The Ultimate Cure,* (Summertown, Tennessee, Book Publishing Company, 2001).

Stormie Omartian, *Greater Health God's Way* (Oregon, Harvest House, 1996).

Taste for Life, January edition, 2007, *Are Plastic Containers Unhealthy?*

www.drwell.com2006; *Plastics Chemicals Alters Female Brain*, Science News, 7/7/06.

Udo Erasmus, *Fats that Health and Fats that Kill* (BC Canada, Alive Books, 1993).

Winter Griffith, M.D *Vitamins, Herbs, Minerals and Supplements* (Cambridge Massachusetts, Da Capo Press, 1998).

ENDNOTES

1   Emilie Barnes and Sue Gregg, *The 15 Minute Meal Planner* (Harvest House, 1994) 238–239.

2   The Mayo Clinic Staff, "Mediterranean diet: Choose this heart-healthy diet option," Mayo Clinic Online, http://www.mayoclinic.com/health/mediterranean-diet/CL00011 (Accessed October 2009).

3   Steve Parker, *The Advanced Mediterranean Diet: Lose Weight, Feel Better, Live Longer* (Gilbert, Arizona: Vanguard Press, 2007), 130.

4   To read the documented research, visit: http://www.oldwayspt.org/med_studies (accessed September, 2013).

5   Steve Meyerowitz, *Water the Ultimate Cure* (Summertwon, TN: Book Publishing Company, 2001) 14.

6   Rietveld A; Wiseman S. Antioxidant effects of tea: evidence from human clinical trials *J Nutr.* 2003; 133(10):3285S–3292S.

7   Fat and Blood, BiblioBazaar, LLC, 2007. Mitchell, S.W., p. 119–154. and The Miracle of Milk—How to Use the Milk Diet Scientifically at Home, Read Books, 2008. McFadden, B.

8   Mattick, E., Golding, J., 1936. Relative value of raw and heated milk in nutrition. Lancet 2:703-6.

9   http://www.msstate.edu/org/fsfa/Vol1/2-Pihlanto.htm. Accessed March 2010.

10   http://www3.interscience.wiley.com/searchallsearch?mode=quicksearch&WISindexid1= WISall&WISsearch1=milk. Accessed March 2010.

11   http://www.foodsci.uoguelph.ca/dairyedu/chem.html and http://www.interscience.wiley.com/journal/119167856/abstract. Accessed March 2010.

12   http://www.pubmedcentral.nih.gov/articlerender.fcgi?artid=128229. Accessed March 2010.

13 Ammendolla, M., Pietrantoni, A., et al, 2007. Bovine lactoferrin inhibits echovirus endocytic pathway by interacting with viral structural peptides. Antiviral Res 73:151-160 and http://www.dairyscience.info/lp-system.htm.

14 http://www.dailymail.co.uk/health/article-399520/Untreated-milk-cuts-childrens-allergies.html. Accessed March 2010.

15 http://journals.cambridge.org/action/display Abstract from Page=onlineandaid=887004. Accessed March 2010.

16 http://jds.fass.org/cgi/reprint/70/1/1 and http://www.springerlink.com/content/u221412 268137476/.

17 http://www3.interscience.wiley.com/journal/119043936/abstract, and Lieverse, R.J., et al, 2006. Role of cholecystokinin in the regulation of satiation and satiety in humans. Ann. New York Acad Sci 713:268-272

18 Dhiman, T. R., et al, 1999. Conjugated linoleic acid content of milk from cows fed different diets. J Dairy Sci 82:2146-56. Accessed March 2010.

19 http://www.foodsci.uoguelph.ca/dairyedu/chem.html#vitamin. Accessed September 2009.

20 Power, M.L., et al, 1999. The role of calcium in health and disease. Am J Obst and Gyn 181:1560 -1569

21 http://content.nejm.org/cgi/content/abstract/328/12/833 (kidney stones). and Nishida, M., et al, 2000. Calcium and the risk for periodontal disease. J Periodontology 71(7):1057-1066. Accessed October 2013.

22 Stevenson, M.A., et al, 2003. Nutrient balance in the diet of spring calving, pasture-fed dairy cows, N Z Vet J 51(2):81-88.

23 http://jds.fass.org/cgi/reprint/56/5/531.

24 Olivecrona, T., et al, "Lipases in Milk" In: Advanced Dairy Chemistry Vol. 1: Proteins 3rd Ed., 473–488, and Shakel-Ur-Rehman, et al, "Indigenous Phosphatases in Milk' In: Advanced Dairy Chemistry Vol. 1: Proteins 3rd Ed., 523–533. And Pruitt, K., 'Lactoperoxidase' In: Advanced Dairy Chemistry Vol. 1: Proteins 3rd Ed., 563–568. Accessed September 2009.

25 http://jds.fass.org/cgi/reprint/79/6/971.

26 de Vrese, M. et al, 2001. Probiotics—compensation for lactase insufficiency. Am J Clin Nutr 73:421S-429s. Accessed September 2013.

27 Dr. Rex Russell, *What the Bible Says About Healthy Living*, (Ventura, CA: Regal Publishing, 1996) 217.

28 Ibid, 219.

29 Patrick J. Bird, Ph.D., "*Grape Juice and Heart Attacks*," University of Florida College of Health and Human Performance Web site: http://www.hhp.ufl.edu/keepingfit. Accessed August 2009.

30 Maroon, Joseph, M.D. *The Longevity Factor*, 2009, 193.

ENDNOTES

31 Rolfes, Sharon, *Understanding Normal and Clinical Nutrition*, 7th ed., 2006 Thomson Wadsworth Publishing, 882.

32 Jacques de Langre, Ph.D. *Sea Salt's Hidden Powers*.

33 Marion Nestle, *What to Eat*, North Point Press.

34 Clinical Nutrition, *A Functional Approach*, 2nd ed., (2004, IFM publishing), 169.

35 Sharon Herbst, *The New Food Lovers Companion*, 2007, Barrons, Educational Series, Inc.

36 Carol Johnston PhD, "Vinegar Helps Lower Blood Glucose," Arizona State University, 2008, http://researchstories.asu.edu/2008/01/vinegar_helps_lower_blood_gluc.html (accessed July, 2009).

37 http://busycooks.about.com/od/quicktips/qt/vinegartips.htm. Accessed July, 2009.

38 Reprinted as a customer service by Clemens Markets, Inc.
The authors are Robert J Price, Ph. D., Seafood Technology Specialist, and Pamela D. Tom, Staff Research Associate, Department of Food Science and Technology, University of California, Davis, California 9516-8598, Publication SG 79/Reprinted October 1985, Oregon State University Extension Service, Oregon State University, Corvallis, Oregon.

39 http://jama.ama-assn.org/cgi/content/full/287/23/3127. Accessed July 2009.

40 Basic H2 is an organic green cleaner sold by Shaklee distributors. You can find a local distributor by contacting our office.

41 Shari Lieberman, Ph.D., *The Real Vitamin and Mineral Book*, 2003 Avery Publishing, 84

42 You can find his research in these books:
How to Live Longer and Feel Better, by Linus Pauling, Ph. D., 1986,
The Healing Factor: Vitamin C against Disease, by Irwin Stone, (Putman 1972)
The Vitamin C Connection, by Emanuel Cheraskin, M.D. (Harper and Row, 1983).
The Clinical Guide to the Use of Vitamin C, edited by Lendon H Smith, M.D., Life Science Press, Tacoma, WA (1988). There are others but too many to give a complete list in this writing.

43 Donald Rudin, M.D. Omega-3 Oils: A Practical Guide (New York, Avery Pub. 1996), 45.

44 Bruce Miller, Dr., *THE AMAZING POWERS OF GARLIC*, Bruce Miller Enterprises.

45 Dr. Miller is the founder of the Diet Analysis Center, Director of Nutrition Research for the American Academy of Nutrition, founder of the publication Health Quest, a member of the Linus Pauling Institute of Science and Medicine and author of 25 books and videos on diet and nutrition, including a book entitled Garlic.

46 Bruce Miller, D.D.S., C.N.S *Protein, A Consumer's Concern*, Bruce Miller's Better Health Series

47 Gemma Gorham, MPH, *Natural Approaches to Prostate Health,* (The Frontrunners, 2005, Wellness Educators LLC).

48 Research contributing to the advancement of understanding aging and the effects of resveratrol and ellagic acid was funded by the National Institutes of Health, and the Glenn Foundation

for Medical Research. David Sinclair, primary research scientist, has been a consultant to Genocea, Shaklee and Sirtris, a GSK company developing sirtuin based drugs. Contributing author to this article was Wayne LaFrance.

49   William Sears, M.D. and Martha Sears, R.N., *The Family Nutrition Book*, 1999 (New York, Little, Brown and Company), 298.

50   Ibid, 306.

51   *Acidosis and Toxicosis are the primary causes of all disease,* http://www.encognitive.com/node/ 1121. Accessed March 2013.

52   Christine Gaber RHN and Charlene Day, RDC, *Why Do I Feel This Way*, 2009 Edition (Ontario, Canada, Health Thru Knowledge Publishing), 31.

53   James L. Wilson, N.D., D.C., Ph.D., *Adrenal Fatigue, the 21st Century Stress Syndrome*, Twelfth Printing, 2008 (Petaluma, CA, Smart Publications), 17.

54   Ibid. 27–45.

55   Gemma Gorham, M.P.H., *Children's Health*, (The Frontrunners publications, Michigan), 2005.

56   Gemma Gorham, M.P.H., *Natural Approaches to Prostate Health*, (The Frontrunners publications, Michigan), 2002.

57   Tori Hudson, N.D., Women's Encyclopedia of Natural Medicine (New York, McGraw Hill, 2008) 55.

58   http://kclibrary.lonestar.edu/decade60.html, Accessed April 2013.

59   http://www.ncbi.nlm.nih.gov/pubmed/9584909?dopt=Abstract, *Triclosan: cytotoxicity, mode of action, and induction of apoptosis in human gingival cells in vitro.* Accessed July 2013.

Zuckerbraun HL, Babich H, May R, Sinensky MC. Accessed October 2013.

60   http://www.ncbi.nlm.nih.gov/pubmed/14996673?dopt=Abstract, *Effect of antibacterial home cleaning and hand washing products on infectious disease symptoms: a randomized, double-blind trial.*

61   Dr.Paula Baile Hamilton, *Toxic Overload,* (New York, Penguin Group), 2005, 104.

62   For full research on fluoride, go to http://www.slweb.org/bibliography.html, this Web site has an extensive list of peer reviewed scientific studies documenting the effects of fluoride on health. There are many opinions on the subject and facts are needed for a solid conclusion. Here are three studies to get you started on this topic: Calderon J, et al. (2000). Influence of fluoride exposure on reaction time and visuospatial organization in children. *Epidemiology* 11(4): S153. Calvert GM, et al. (1998). Health effects associated with sulfuryl fluoride and methyl bromide exposure among structural fumigation workers. *American Journal of Public Health* 88(12):1774-80. Ekambaram P, Paul V. (2001). Calcium preventing locomotor behavioral and dental toxicities of fluoride by decreasing serum fluoride level in rats. *Environmental Toxicology and Pharmacology* 9(4):141-146. Li XS. (1995). Effect of fluoride exposure on intelligence in children. *Fluoride* 28(4):189-192.

INDEX

ABOUT THE AUTHORS

Annette Reeder is the founder of Designed Healthy Living (a source for answers to biblical health and consultations) and author of *Healthy Treasures Cookbook* and *Treasures of Healthy Living Bible Study*. Annette has her B.S. in Nutrition and Biblical Studies and is a graduate of Liberty University; but her greatest training has come from being a wife, mother, and caregiver for over twenty-five years. Her career as a Biblical Nutrition Consultant allows her the blessings of seeing lives changed as people apply Scripture to their physical, emotional, and spiritual health. Annette loves the Lord and continually thanks God for the treasures that come from His Word. She eagerly and generously shares her personal journey into God's truths and treasures.

Dr. Richard (Dick) Couey is professor emeritus of health sciences at Baylor University in Waco, Texas. His areas of specialty are human physiology, human anatomy, sports medicine, and nutrition. He is a former member of the President's Commission on Physical Fitness and Sports, and he served as exercise physiology consultant for the US Olympic Team. Prior to coming to Baylor, he was a pitcher in the Chicago Cubs Organization. Dr Couey was educated at Baylor (B.A.), Sam Houston State University (M.A.), and Texas A&M University (Ph.D.). He has written and published over twenty books on subjects that include nutrition, physical fitness, wellness, and enzymes. He has spoken in over 300 churches throughout the US and internationally on "Why Christians Should Care for Their Temple (body)." His hobbies include working out, serving as a Deacon at his church, and golfing.

OTHER BOOKS AND MATERIALS
BY ANNETTE AND DR. RICHARD COUEY:

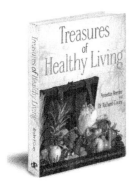

Treasures of Healthy Living

Everyone loves a treasure hunt. The hunt can be almost as rewarding as the final treasure! Follow the clues on our map and discover the answers to a healthy life full of vitality. This study will unveil the counterfeits and substitutions currently robbing us of energy and zest for living. Then it will fill the void with overflowing riches of health. This Bible Study will give you and your group the tools needed to reclaim health in the balance God designed. This study speaks to a new generation hungry for answers and looking for God's design.

Available soft cover and Kindle

Healthy Treasures Cookbook

This bounty of recipes and cooking tips will encourage you to bring healthy treasures back to the dinner table. Surprise and delight will abound as you please your family with these tasty meals that will also contribute to their health and well-being. Whether you are a beginner or novice in the kitchen, this book covers it all.

Available soft cover

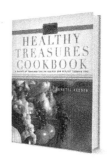

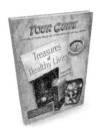

Tour Guide

Building upon the message of Annette Reeder and Dr. Richard Couey in the Treasures *of Healthy Living Bible* study, this *Tour Guide* will enhance all groups' experience as they delve into the treasure hunt. This guide is full of tips on food ideas, teaching options and in-depth review, anyone can lead a class, Book Club or small group with this valuable resource. Designed to bring women, men, couples and families back to the dinner table showcasing God's richest foods and back to a relationship with God that encompasses all areas of their life.

Available in soft cover and e-book download.

Daniel Fast

Fasting made simple with this complete resource with guidelines, menu plans, recipes, testimonies, journal pages and daily devotions. Available as download on website and Kindle

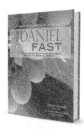

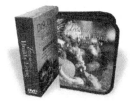

The DVD series will enhance the Treasures of Healthy Living Bible study with lessons on topics such as Inflammation, Antioxidants, Heart Health, Spiritual Health, Immune Health, Protecting Your Mind, Mindless Eating, plus creative tips on cooking with fresh herbs, making the real bread and overlooked topics such as forgiveness.

These DVDs with over 12 hours of health living teachings will greatly improve your understanding of God's design of your body for His kingdom.

Books, DVDs and other materials for sale at www.DesignedHealthyLiving.com

Designed Healthy Living

Changing lives one meal at a time.

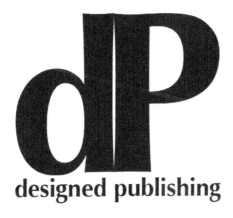

designed publishing

Designed Publishing Since 2004

Designed Healthy Living

Glen Allen, Virginia

804-798-6565

www.designedhealthyliving.com

Email: yourfriends@designedhealthyliving.com

CPSIA information can be obtained at www.ICGtesting.com
Printed in the USA
BVOW09s1952070915

416774BV00003B/34/P